# Creative Expressive Activities
# and Asperger's Syndrome
## Social and Emotional Skills and Positive Life
## Goals for Adolescents and Young Adults

*Judith Martinovich*

Jessica Kingsley Publishers
London and Philadelphia

First published in 2006
by Jessica Kingsley Publishers
116 Pentonville Road
London N1 9JB, UK
and
400 Market Street, Suite 400
Philadelphia, PA 19106, USA

www.jkp.com

Coventry University

**Library of Congress Cataloging in Publication Data**
Martinovich, Judith, 1955-
    Creative expressive activities and Asperger's syndrome : social and emotional skills and positive life goals for adolescents and young adults / Judith Martinovich.
        p. cm.
    Includes bibliographical references and index.
    ISBN-13: 978-1-84310-812-2 (pbk. : alk. paper)
    ISBN-10: 1-84310-812-7 (pbk. : alk. paper)   1.  Asperger's syndrome—Patients—Education. 2. Asperger's syndrome—Social aspects. 3. Creative ability. I. Title.
    RJ506.A9M376 2005
    618.92'858832—dc22

                                                    2005014168


**British Library Cataloguing in Publication Data**
A CIP catalogue record for this book is available from the British Library

ISBN-13: 978 1 84310 812 2
ISBN-10: 1 84310 812 7


Printed and Bound in Great Britain by
Athenaeum Press, Gateshead, Tyne and Wear

Chris, Anna, Sam

With love

# Acknowledgements

With appreciation to Warren and Joan Moore, my parents, whose support and encouragement of lifelong learning allowed this book to come together from many directions and experiences over a period of years; Tony Attwood for his diagnosis skills, the beginning; Eve Thalor and Jeanne Marron of West Bergen Center for Child and Youth for sharing their work with so many people, including myself; and the many children and adults with Asperger's Syndrome, for their purity of spirit.

# Contents

# List of figures

# List of creative activities

# Preface

Young people with Asperger's Syndrome have concerns similar to their peers – transitions, independence, decisions and relationships. Asperger traits are likely to be less obvious in adolescence than in childhood due to increasingly modified behavior. Yet the individual with Asperger's is likely to feel more isolated and be more susceptible to depression than his peers.

Support of the whole person is important. People with Asperger's Syndrome are wonderful individuals, each exceptional in their own way, typically with good hearts and integrity, sometimes eccentric but with unique skills and enormous potential to make their own lives and the lives of other people around them extraordinary.

Perhaps the greatest need for the adolescent is to make meaningful connections with other people, to feel they have something meaningful to offer and have skills to make positive choices about their future. Activities in this book are structured to address these and many other issues. Problematic AS traits are a reason to look for support but provide a weak, non-affirming core for support and/or a support group.

The most effective and engaging support is in opportunities for social interaction, genuine affirmation and exploration of the whole person, their individuality, potential, and strengths. These are the objectives and goals of activities in this book – individualized therapy within a group context – activities that address AS traits while affirming individual exploration and expression:

1. Adolescents and young people with Asperger's Syndrome have different needs to the child in grade school. They are developing a distinctive identity and this book takes a *positive and broad* approach to support and development of the *whole person*. It is a *wellness model*, engaging individuals in their own development with a *creative, visual, and experiential "language"* suited to the Asperger way of thinking.

2.   Creative activities and interventions are grounded in contemporary principles of *Positive Psychology* and *Social and Emotional Learning* – principles for building long-term satisfaction, happiness, and psychological resilience.

3.   There is a *broad, comprehensive approach* to Asperger traits including work with cognitive processing, personal development, and social synchrony; and introducing *different therapies* that can be applied to Asperger's Syndrome.

4.   Activities are designed to *adapt* to different ages and skill levels; individual or group; school or psychological setting; available time and space; *with or without Asperger's.*

5.   *Creative activities are multidimensional.* They complement and reinforce each other in support of the whole person. This book includes activities in art, music, dance, movement, drama, yoga and relaxation, and cognitive and behavioral skills.

If you work or live with Asperger's Syndrome and you have creative ideas that contribute to positive development, resilience, and strengths, we would love to hear from you. Please contact Judith Martinovich at JRM@creativeexpressiveactivities.com.

# Part I

# A Multidimensional Approach to Asperger's Syndrome

# CHAPTER 1

# Introduction

This book is written within a framework of principles known to contribute to a happy life and resilient person. It is a framework that considers the whole person and is relevant to the support of all young people, with and without Asperger's Syndrome (Chapter 2). Against that framework, typical AS traits are discussed and how they may affect general principles of healthy development (Chapter 3). AS traits can be used as strengths, not just perceived as weaknesses, and activities are introduced which apply or modify them accordingly. With knowledge and awareness, people with AS can do a great deal to turn a diagnosis around to work for them, not against them.

## A multifaceted approach to Asperger support strategies

1. Individuals are multifaceted – Asperger's Syndrome adds to the complexity with its pattern of traits, differing between individuals.

2. Comprehensive strategies for supporting positive development should have many dimensions.

3. Creative activities are multidimensional and multisensory and offer support strategies to suit individual differences.

During formative and maturing stages of life, important choices are made and self-concept evolves. Difficulties may appear to be situation specific – adolescent issues, school performance, relationships. Yet the outcome of these experiences is likely to have far-reaching consequences on health and happiness. The AS person needs support that considers the whole person and that develops self-knowledge, useful tools, and strategies.

Most people experience traits characteristic of Asperger's Syndrome to some degree (the definition of Asperger's Syndrome and an explanation of its traits can be found in Chapter 3). Obsessive interests, social difficulties, verbal clumsiness, and difficulties with organization are traits commonly experienced. When one or more of those traits causes difficulty in functioning in some aspect of life, support is needed for modification.

Yet it is the less obvious traits that have the most impact. A focus on modification of behavior often overlooks difficulties in conceptual thinking, goal setting, problem solving, difficulty in articulating thoughts, lack of self-consciousness and understanding of complex emotions, and difficulties with gross and fine motor skills. The positive characteristics of Asperger's Syndrome and individual strengths are rarely given credit. The best support will consider the many dimensions of the individual with Asperger's Syndrome and use a multifaceted approach to treatment.

Although certain criteria must be met for a diagnosis of Asperger's Syndrome, the patterns vary enormously. One person with traits of Asperger's Syndrome may need help with social skills; another person may cope very well indeed without formal assistance, and life experience is likely to modify their traits over time to the degree that Asperger's Syndrome is barely perceptible. Identifying and addressing specific areas according to the individual's experience is more useful than a generalized, single dimensional approach.

People with Asperger's Syndrome typically receive, process, and learn information in non-conventional ways. That is a motivating force for writing this book. Many AS people are more receptive to information when it is experienced visually. Some have an adverse reaction to the parent or teacher who believes that if something is repeated often enough or loud enough, the child will eventually "get it." For the AS individual, noise or repetition of complex information may be overwhelming. The consequence is likely to be withdrawal or a meltdown. Relating information in ways that engage the person and meet their needs for processing is a fundamental step to effective support.

People with Asperger's Syndrome can be brilliant – in their own Asperger type of way. In other areas they can flounder. There is often a weakness in semantics and pragmatics – verbal gymnastics for an AS individual. Despite that, many treatment and educational programs teach social skills in ways that are presented verbally. This is tantamount to teaching a second language in the language that is being taught. The strategy is repetition until the listener remembers. Children and adolescents may feel stupid because even if they remember, they can't apply what they've been taught. It's useful to integrate non-verbal strategies congruent with the AS way of thinking, to facilitate effective learning. Goals are to build and strengthen neural pathways for new behavior. Verbal and non-verbal strategies through multifaceted interventions will reinforce each other.

Ideally, the individual is a cooperative partner in the learning process. There should be a reciprocal aspect to the relationship. The AS individual can teach the parent or professional how they think and what they feel – the Asperger perspective is just as valid as the non-Asperger perspective. The parent or professional can help the individual understand the benefit of activities and provide an environment that is engaging and motivating. Reciprocity relies on individual and professional sharing a language that facilitates communication. Art provides a means for genuine, expressive communication without the narrow constraints of conventional language.

Asperger's Syndrome is a pervasive developmental disorder. Support goals are not to cure but to modify behavior. Goals and treatment often focus on modifying social and study skills, appropriate language and behavior, respect for others' space, maintaining eye contact, organization of schoolwork, and self-regulation of emotions. These are important skills for completing an education and interacting well with peers. But if they utilize cognitive and behavioral strategies almost exclusively, they will fail to address the underlying AS traits and processing abilities which have an impact on other important aspects of development.

The need for problem solving and social skills may be obvious and attended to by alert parents and teachers. The inner confusion and self-doubt may not be so easily detected or addressed. Before diagnosis, many young AS individuals know instinctively that they are "different" and struggle to appear to be normal. The continual effort to understand the non-Asperger way of doing things can be confusing and tiring. To cope, many individuals adopt avoidance strategies, resulting in problems not being addressed and potential not being realized. At the same time a negative concept of self-esteem evolves.

Without an understanding of their own potential, choices in life may be designed to cater to restricting Asperger characteristics ("I don't want to join a club because it's difficult to talk to other people") rather than Asperger strengths and characteristics that could be used to reach life goals ("I wonder if anyone else in this school is interested in Star Trek"). The best strategy to help AS individuals supports the whole person, not just outstanding traits. The best support strategies will help them know themselves a little better, in an environment that affirms individuality and uniqueness. As a result, they will have knowledge and confidence in their own strengths and ability to draw on their own resources. Creative activities affirm individual strengths which, in turn, lead to increased resilience.

## How can this book help a person with Asperger's Syndrome?

This book offers a broad therapeutic approach. Cognitive and behavioral therapies are effective and necessary. However, this book integrates cognitive behavioral techniques with alternative ways of learning and processing which are often non-verbal and congruent with the Asperger way of thinking. Attention is given to the inner feelings and experience of the individual, and their connection to choices, behavior, and goals. The overall framework gives cohesiveness to support strategies, while introducing activities designed to meet personal needs and address individual differences.

This book is ideal for individuals who prefer a visual and experiential learning style. Typically, AS individuals have difficulty grasping concepts, linking ideas, and seeing the whole picture. They are more likely to see the world through personal experience, literal interpretation, and learned rules. Many – although not all – learn and understand in pictures better than words and concepts. Temple Grandin, who wrote a first-person account about Asperger's Syndrome titled *Thinking in Pictures* (1995), has been innovative in her scientific field of expertise because of her visual and experiential approach (taking the visual perspective of the animals she was working with) rather than a purely intellectual approach.

Albert Einstein had traits characteristic of Asperger's Syndrome. In some ways he exhibited a child-like naivety with simple concepts. In his later years he was invited with his wife to visit a movie studio to see a movie being made. He was fascinated and delighted with the idea that he could sit in a stationary car with a filmed backdrop of moving scenery, with the end result that the car appeared to be moving on film. The concept had not occurred to him until he actually saw it. Einstein's own genius and superior insights were based on combinations of mental images, for which he then had to find a verbal language to communicate his ideas to other people. For example, the initial revelation about relativity came to him as he imagined himself riding a beam of light and looking back at a church steeple.

A concept is an idea, often abstract or not fully formulated, general in nature rather than specific, and a starting point from which assumptions can be made to further its understanding. A concept might relate to friendship (principles of sharing) or social skills (importance of good manners) or the reasoning behind a parent's attitude (she tends to raise her voice when she has a lot to do). An AS child might see a series of events but is unable to make a connection between them (Mom is yelling again – why?). Conceptual thinking allows generalizations and connections to be made. It is essential to personal and intellectual development.

Through different processes – in our case, creative processes such as storytelling and art-making – connections can be made to a bigger picture. Experiences can be seen as part of a greater whole, not just isolated pieces of information. Patterns and structures can be identified, making associations and allowing generalizations and abstract conceptual possibilities.

Thinking visually allows development of a complementary language. This has positive implications for communication, understanding self, and being able to share perspectives, fears, and dreams. Through visual imagery, imaginative and innovative thought can be stimulated. Unique connections can be made. Instead of restricting emotions to inadequate concrete terms, creative activities offer a comprehensive and expressive language.

As with anything else, the more something is practiced, the more neurological connections develop to strengthen that area of the brain. Creative activities such as those introduced in this book are multidimensional, complementing and reinforcing each other, integrated in a multifaceted bigger picture. Creative activities provide variety and opportunities for self-expression that lean more to learning through leisure than formal learning, making ongoing support interventions more engaging. They also offer a variety of other benefits including practice of motor skills, building relationships within groups, articulating thoughts, and participants being valued for the unique contribution they have to make.

## Overview and structure of book

### Part I

A fundamental goal in child and adolescent support – with or without Asperger's Syndrome – is building core skills and strengths toward a foundation for potential to be realized. This book addresses AS traits with that goal. The goals of different activities contribute to the whole person and their positive, resilient personal development.

Parents and professionals cannot predict or prevent all of the potentially harmful life experiences that may be encountered. A more useful strategy is to develop the inner resources to draw on in unique or difficult circumstances – resources that include resilience and a framework for making positive choices.

Chapter 2 summarizes those things which research has shown contribute to resilience and a happy, fulfilled life. The importance of goals and signature strengths is a focus of Positive Psychology. Competence in Social and Emotional Learning (SEL) is required for effective interaction with the world and in achievement of goals.

Chapter 3 identifies the nature of Asperger's Syndrome and how it is likely to impact on healthy development. Support strategies are discussed in ways that can be tailored to meet individual needs. The areas relevant to AS are basically broken down into three broad components, drawn from the Positive Psychology and SEL framework:

- conceptual thought processes and cognitive processing difficulties
- self-awareness and self-related skills
- social skills and "connectedness."

## CONCEPTUAL THOUGHT PROCESSES AND COGNITIVE PROCESSING DIFFICULTIES

AS individuals have a tendency toward concrete thought and literal interpretation, leading to difficulties with problem solving and influencing every part of their lives. Conceptual thinking allows us to consider alternative perspectives and options in a given situation, including understanding that other people may have a different perspective. Being able to think abstractly or conceptually is vitally important to furthering education, learning life skills, learning from experience, and being able to set goals and make plans. AS thought processing may also cause language skills to be impaired because of semantic and pragmatic weaknesses.

## SELF-AWARENESS AND SELF-RELATED SKILLS

Emotion experienced by the AS individual is not always understood well or expressed appropriately. Depression is more commonly experienced by AS adolescents than by non-Asperger peers. Anxiety, depression, confidence, esteem and emotional self-regulation issues are interconnected and can impact greatly on adolescent development. Confounding this, motor and sensory integration issues can cause problems with distractibility and impulse control.

## SOCIAL SKILLS AND "CONNECTEDNESS"

Interpersonal skills are greatly influenced by cognitive processing and attitude toward self. The importance of making emotional connections for developing a healthy and happy life cannot be underestimated. There is a great amount of evidence that having an active connection to a larger social network is important to physical and mental health. Emotionally expressive connections to interests beyond one's self also make a positive contribution to well-being. Disconnectedness is a fundamental issue that can cause lifelong difficulties for the AS individual – in education, at work, and in personal relationships. Awareness and strategies in this area are very important to positive development.

## Part II

Part II introduces creative activities that can be used in a treatment program and modified to meet the unique needs of an individual. Chapter 2 summarizes principles that have been shown to contribute to positive adolescent development. The activities in Part II are designed to integrate that information with typical AS characteristics and personal needs. Thus, the creative activities and ideas suggested in the remainder of the book focus on areas that include the following:

- importance of a positive and complex (many faceted) self-knowledge and self-concept
- understanding of unique strengths and how to utilize them
- acknowledging, clarifying, and coping with emotions
- importance of relationships and "connectedness" and skills to facilitate "connectedness"
- being able to think and work conceptually and abstractly
- skills to adapt to demands and expectations of a variety of environments
- problem solving skills, adaptability, and resilience in the face of difficulties and setbacks
- ability to positively handle transitions and change.

The general goal of the activities in Part II is to build a positive and resourceful young adult. While traditional cognitive and behavioral strategies are used, there is an emphasis on activities that enhance skills and focus on self-knowledge, resilience, and development, but with a recreational flavor. It is intended that this book takes some of the "hard" out of learning and helps individuals with AS, their parents, and therapists to recognize and integrate therapeutic opportunities in informal and everyday situations. It serves as an introduction to various specialized areas.

Adolescents and young adults with Asperger's Syndrome present unique challenges for parents and professionals. A new set of issues is emerging – often related to relationships, need for conceptual thinking, decision making, and self-concept. These issues may not be as distinct as they were in younger years and the teenager finds himself or herself too busy to attend groups that they don't enjoy, in which they are not engaged and for which they see no benefit. Indeed, they are busy, and groups have to be enjoyable and produce results or members will not be retained. An advantage of groups based on the type of activities in this book is that the concept of a leisure or social group can be promoted, rather than a purely therapeutic, educational group.

Diverse activities are brought together offering a choice to suit individual ability. It is useful to focus on specific needs rather than a broad diagnosis. Some of the strategies suggested here will not suit all AS individuals. Some of the activities will be very suitable for ADHD individuals or individuals with no diagnosis at all – simply as an additional teaching activity.

An objective of creative and novel interventions is to broaden the methods of processing information through multisensory and multimodal stimulation and experience. Sensory integration is the therapeutic approach of integrating the visual, auditory, touching, taste, and smell senses. In addition there is the integration of the proprioception sense, awareness of the body and its movements. A most natural way to integrate all of these senses is through play and creative opportunities.

Different modes of learning, including play, contribute to increasing complexity, use of different areas of the brain, stimulating and modifying neural pathways and integrating skills. Creative and complementary therapies generate new ways of looking at things, processing information and learning strategies. Familiar boundaries are removed, integrative and adaptive skills learned, and choices and potential explored. It is hoped that the parent, teacher, and therapist will use the basic principles to devise their own therapeutic activities – and enjoy the creative process too!

In a nutshell, "therapy" in this book is not confined to cognitive and behavioral techniques. It integrates multisensory, multidimensional strategies to reveal, explore, and express individuality and develop different ways of thinking. Therapy should not have to be all hard work. It is my hope that this book helps the individual with Asperger's Syndrome to dream a little, and find ways to make the dreams come true.

# CHAPTER 2

# What makes an adaptive, resilient, and happy person?

There is rarely a time in anyone's life when there is a sense that their potential has been fulfilled. Life continues to present new challenges and unexpected twists and turns. What is usually fairly constant, however, is the attitude with which each of us perceives life events and makes our choices. Although each may seem small in itself, our attitude and choices all contribute to a larger pattern of lifelong goals and direction.

Childhood is a time of dependency and concrete thinking, when assumptions and perspectives are quietly acquired through experience. During adolescence that experience is expanded through growing independence, transitions, opportunities and frustration, leaps in growth, and bouts of self-doubt and confusion. The individual's world view and attitudes are often challenged at a time when important choices have to be made. This chapter presents contemporary research that offers useful information in supporting an individual during that time.

Research in education, psychology, language, and related fields has helped identify conditions which help ease the path and build a foundation for a happy, healthy adulthood. Yet with so much specialized knowledge, it can be a challenge to select appropriate information from the broad and comprehensive body of knowledge available. The activities in Part II draw on an eclectic mix of theories:

1.  Behavioral theory is highly appropriate for the concrete and literal tendencies of an AS individual and particularly useful in modifying social skills in younger people. Practice and reward increases desired behavior.

2.  Social learning theory explains how a child learns behavior through observation of others at school and home; and how new behaviors can be learned through "modeling" in group or a therapeutic environment.

3.  Cognitive restructuring – or teasing apart and refuting habitual ways of thinking about ourselves and events in our lives – is extremely important, especially for people who can be narrow in perspective and not fully understand that other people have different and valid perspectives of the same event.

4.  Gestalt theory includes techniques such as drama and role playing to increase awareness of the "big picture," and integration of feelings.

5.  Family counseling is useful because it is typically some time before an AS individual becomes independent. Development of the individual has a significant impact on family dynamics, and family dynamics impact on individual development. As the individual matures there may also be practical problems in achieving independence which can be addressed through family counseling.

6.  Reality theory is a very rational and goal/activity oriented approach that draws on strengths and provides structure for increased responsibility and ongoing decision making.

7.  Moral development and ability to develop personal meaning are also important. Although AS individuals are typically not "bad," they may need to clarify a value system for themselves for self-directed guidance, especially to build resilience against alienation or depression.

Techniques from all of these areas and theories should be used when appropriate. However, the goal of positive support has led this book to focus on a couple of theoretical models in particular. A basic framework is provided by some of the principles of *Positive Psychology*. These principles are supported and complemented by the educationally motivated *Social and Emotional Learning* (SEL) approach. Positive Psychology and SEL provide relevant, recently researched, positive, and practical structures. Understanding a little about these underlying theories allows parents and professionals to have clear goals yet be adaptive in clinical and non-clinical interaction with the adolescent. The Positive Psychology and SEL models emphasize skills that include:

- positive perceptions of self and potential
- fulfilling and resilient happiness
- being able to employ social and emotional skills in the quest to connect to others.

Positive Psychology focuses on identifying and developing strengths and has a goal-task orientation which suits the concrete thinking of the AS individual. Social and Emotional Learning focuses on the personal and social skills and tools that are necessary for effective negotiation through life. This is not to say that other methodologies don't have useful information to offer parents and professionals, but the Positive Psychology and SEL models represent and justify a practical approach to our goal – capable, happy, and resilient maturity.

From these principles, a useful framework for individualized intervention is presented. It can be used by parents and professionals – teachers, therapists, psychologists, counselors, social workers. *Exercises are focused primarily at the adolescent level but can sensibly be simplified for younger, precocious children or modified for adults.*

## Positive Psychology

The term Positive Psychology was coined comparatively recently for a model of psychology directed toward enhancing happiness and emotional resilience. It is supported by the work of Alfred Adler, Abraham Maslow, Carl Rogers, Carl Jung, and theorists who focus on psychological well-being and development of potential. Behavioral and cognitive interventions are also used in Positive Psychology. A major proponent of Positive Psychology has been Martin Seligman.

Most psychological models operate from the position of reducing the symptoms of mental illness and disorders. Positive Psychology considers positive thoughts and emotions to be the foundation of a healthy mental life, not just the result, and they should be given the same or more importance as negative thoughts and emotions. In addition, positive emotions have a function above and beyond just feeling good. They increase intellectual and physical performance. They provide a foundation for resilience.

## *"Are you happy yet?"*

### THE NATURE OF HAPPINESS

Considering that happiness is an implicit goal for most people, parents, and professionals, it is surprising how little is known about it – how to identify it, how to develop it, how to sustain it. Most parents would like their children to be happy. It is generally assumed that a good education, job, and financial security will go a long way to success and subsequent happiness. Consequently, much of adolescence is directed to achieve this end. Yet in his research on what it is that makes a happy life, Mihaly Csikszentmihalyi (1997) noted that a barely literate but proficient factory worker can be as happy as or happier than a high achieving CEO or Nobel Prize winner.

Money, fame, and associated symbols of success have a weak association with how happy people perceive themselves to be. Changes in circumstance (getting a promotion, winning the lottery, or losing a lot of money, even failing health) may have an immediate effect but it is relatively short lived. The individual will adapt quickly and the original level of happiness will generally return. The greatest exception to this is the longer term effect of losing someone or something well loved.

We are born with a certain inclination toward happiness or sadness, optimism or pessimism, and these will bias choices and reactions throughout life. People often have a picture or story in their head of how happy they are, or how happy they believe they should be, and will fit the evidence to that picture. Consequently, their assessment of how happy they are is relatively fixed according to the picture or the story.

Knowing this serves two purposes. First, the happiness that people rate themselves as having may not be a realistic indicator of the quality of their life. Second, if the story they tell themselves is more useful in determining happiness or contentment than events and circumstances, realizing and modifying thoughts about life and events is a key to therapeutic interventions.

A common measurement of happiness is the emotion most evident at any given moment, which usually reflects the activity at the time. A response to "How are you feeling?" is likely to be based on an assessment of the most salient emotions. Yet a person who is generally happy may cry while watching a sad movie, be extremely excited at a baseball game, or disappointed.

If identified through reactive emotions, happiness is a transitory and vulnerable emotional state of being. It is largely dependent on other people and external conditions. The desire for this type of happiness can result in a search for repetitive exciting or pleasurable experiences. It is not resilient.

To help adolescents develop strategies for an intrinsically happy and resilient life, it is necessary to know the nature of happiness and what makes people happy. In his book *Authentic Happiness*, Martin Seligman (2002) makes the distinction between:

- happiness characterized by transient feelings and emotions, based on experience or external stimulation with little genuine connection to the person experiencing them other than their emotional reaction

- happiness that is authentic because it is derived from the "exercise of strengths" and character, a realization of personal potential, engaging and affirming the individual.

The first type of happiness is experienced with positive feelings and contributes to a "pleasant" life. Conditions that produce positive emotions are often based on sensory reaction such as enjoying good food or being an audience member in a theater. Although not a deep-seated happiness, these feelings can be instrumental in increasing the creativity of an individual, and their ability to learn and adapt. For example, a liked teacher and pleasant learning environment will result in more receptivity than a disliked teacher and uncomfortable classroom, no matter how capable the teacher is.

The second type of happiness is not experienced in terms of fleeting feelings and emotions. It is the sense of fulfillment derived from challenge and exercise of using personal character, strengths, and control towards completion of a goal. In that process, self-consciousness and time can be lost. A sense of integration and "flow" may be achieved and the result is "gratification" – a more authentic and resilient fulfillment than happiness from momentary pleasures or external conditions.

Gratification is the satisfaction that a mother or chef might derive from cooking food that meets personal standards. In a restaurant, a chef may use skill, creativity, and service to present a meal that leaves him satisfied with a job well done. A mother may develop recipes of nutritional food for her children, putting in more effort than a frozen meal would require, but congruent with her values of being a good mother. This is the kind of satisfaction an actor in the theater might achieve from utilizing his potential, meeting the challenge of a difficult play or audience, "losing himself" in the performance, learning and growing from the experience.

Ideally, a full life will have a mixture of happy feelings that come from pleasant experiences and a deeper measure of contentment from meeting challenges and utilizing potential.

*Removing unhappiness does not make happiness*

Parents and supporting professionals are usually motivated to reduce or remove negative emotions (depression, pessimism, sadness) and conditions that may set up negative emotions. Little professional attention has been given to enhancing positive emotions for their own sake, almost as though it is expected that positive emotions will happen by accident or default after negative emotions have been removed. This is akin to making the effort to take time off for a vacation but making no plans to use that vacation time. But positive emotions have significant power of their own and pursuit of positive emotions is a goal well justified.

Positive emotions are foundation building blocks for development, even having a positive impact on physical health. They dissipate negative emotions and, through them, a person is better able and equipped to meet challenges, learn and adapt (Seligman 2002). "Social emotional capacities" have been shown to affect or determine ability to listen and communicate, concentrate, recognize, understand, solve problems, cooperate, self-motivation, and conflict resolution (Cohen 2001). In fact, positive emotions are so influential in the healthy development of children, it is just as important to nurture positive emotions for their influence as it is to reduce negative emotions for their less desirable impact.

The work of Barbara Fredrickson (1998, 2001) has shown that while experiencing positive emotions, an individual has great advantages. While in a positive mood, there is increased creativity and generative thought, more openness to ideas, learning, and social interaction, and a tenacity and thoroughness to problem solving. A happy outlook is also associated with better health, endurance of pain and longer life, generative playfulness and productivity, selection of higher goals, better performance, and tenacity in achieving goals. In general, positive emotions help set the stage for potential of the adolescent to be developed, with long-term effects.

In *Authentic Happiness* (2002), Seligman writes: "Positive emotion has consequences that broaden and build intellectual, social and physical resources that are the bank accounts for your children to draw upon later in life." With that in mind, developing a framework for being happy should not be seen as an indulgence but an essential part of treatment planning and support for any individual. Being happy promotes positive choices; positive choices enhance the chances of being happy.

Most adolescents can write a shopping list a mile long of things that make them feel happy. Contemporary adolescents live in a world with an abundance of opportunities to satisfy sight, touch, taste, and other senses. Homes are equipped with machines that instantly produce music, movies, food, and an endless variety of pleasures. Unfortunately, the fleeting nature of these pleasures can result in a need to habitually seek out instant gratification. When the senses have been satisfied, a feeling of boredom can set in.

We now focus our attention on opportunities to experience more enduring happiness – gratification, feeling good rather than happy. The experience of deeper satisfaction has been written about extensively by Csikszentmihalyi (1990, 1996, 1997; Csikzentmihalyi and Csikzentmihalyi 1988; Csikzentmihalyi, Rathunde and Whalen 1997). His research has found that there are some activities which engage the skills of an individual in a challenging yet rewarding manner, resulting in a loss of self-consciousness and experience of a state of "flow." Flow produces a relaxed alertness and energy, resulting from an activity that is challenging but achievable. Time can pass without awareness and consciousness of self lost.

Living a life that engages the individual in challenging activities maximizes opportunities for authentic satisfaction. It increases a sense of accomplishment, offering resilience and some autonomy from the influences of life events. These activities or interests may not be perceived as particularly valuable in themselves yet they offer a buffer to feelings of depression so common for adolescents, and particularly common for adolescents with Asperger's Syndrome. The following example given by Csikszentmihalyi (1997) illustrates the significant impact on mental health that such activities can have.

A chronic schizophrenic who had been hospitalized for ten years was happiest and most motivated when doing her nails. Hospital staff developed that small interest with an opportunity to learn skills of the trade with a professional manicurist. The patient's health and autonomy improved so dramatically that within a year she developed from taking care of the nails of other patients to being back in the community, under supervision, with her own small business.

The implicit goal of support is to "empower" the individual. Yet the positive influence of challenging, satisfying activities has not been given a great deal of attention. In earlier times, an adolescent came to maturity through ritual or partaking in adult activities which proved his maturity in concrete ways. In the twenty-first century young people are likely to celebrate their maturity with a party or a new car. Reward with little personal effort is not likely to be empowering.

Evidence from the "happiness research" suggests that there is more benefit in playing a guitar than listening to a CD, learning to sail a boat or ski rather than watching sailing or skiing on television; taking part in local activities, clubs, sport events, mentoring opportunities, building and developing skills, producing and contributing to something rather than being passively entertained. Opportunities to employ and develop personal strengths provide opportunities to feel valuable and valued.

More directly, opportunities that utilize personal strengths and skills in a challenging way are likely to produce the gratification identified by Csikszentmihalyi. Gus the Grocer who does his work with little interest is not as likely to be as satisfied as Tom the Trainee who goes out of his way to be helpful to customers and designs more interesting product displays, an activity for which he has the skills but still poses an engaging challenge.

Helping adolescents find ways to develop skills and meet personal challenges has enormous implications from a therapeutic perspective. Approaching therapy from an "illness model," we help adolescents eliminate immediate problems with an assumption that a happy life will fill the vacuum. (When the bullying at school is stopped, Sean will be happy.)

Integrating opportunities into therapy that include positive, challenging, and satisfying goals is just as important as dealing with issues such as the bullying at school. Identifying and encouraging the engagement of personal strengths, particularly in flow activities, will contribute to development of a healthy and resilient adolescent.

### No man is an island: importance of connectedness

There is a tendency for contemporary society and psychology to focus on the individual. When Martin Seligman introduced the concept of Positive Psychology, he attributed the rise in contemporary adolescent violence and depression to an "I–We" imbalance. There is an overemphasis on self-esteem and tendency for adolescents to blame everything but themselves for things that go wrong in their lives. These factors combine to make a "brittle generation," equating life satisfaction with individual success or failure. Adolescents often feel disconnected – from their schools, their parents, their friends. Yet feeling connected to a "bigger picture" has an important contribution to make in development of resilience.

Much of our identity is defined by our relationships and the influence of family, society, and culture. We spend roughly one-third of the day alone – more than in traditional societies – but the greatest personal growth for the adolescent will occur in the other two-thirds because it is in the context of interaction with other people that social learning takes place, risks are taken, and challenges resolved (Csikszentmihalyi 1997).

There is a strong association between being with other people and increased happiness. In the company of others, we focus more on them, and less on ourselves and our own thoughts. There tends to be more negative thinking when we are alone. An effort may be made toward positive mood for other people that would not be made for ourselves on our own. Opportunities for connectedness with others offer a valuable source of support for individuals with Asperger's Syndrome to grow.

Genuine connectedness shares some characteristics with flow activities. Personal skills are used and there is an implicit goal–feedback loop in interaction with other people, characteristic of flow activities. Our goal is to communicate with others and we are rewarded with their attention and reciprocated effort. It is particularly satisfying if our conversations are challenging and allow authentic self-expression. In the most beneficial relationships, the individual plays a contributing part of a greater whole, and the whole is partially determined by the contribution made by the individual.

Being meaningfully connected to a group or body larger than ourselves makes an important contribution to identity and self-concept. The confidence and esteem for the culturally connected adolescent is protected and nurtured when he can draw on the strength of the larger group ("I'm not just Mike – I'm an American"). The adolescent who does voluntary work may feel a sense of gratitude or flow, or there may be support through the companionship of like-minded people, and feelings of being useful.

There is a significant association between a complex (many faceted) self-concept and resilience. If a person's self-concept is based on two or three facets – student, daughter, friend – and then the friend moves away, the self-concept is severely shaken. When the self-concept is more complex (student, a circle of friends at church, another group at school, an active interest in exotic fish, a Trekkie who goes to Star Trek conventions and emails other Trekkies) there will be more resilience in the face of losing a friend.

A distinction must be made between the qualities of belonging (as a group member) and connectedness (an experience where the individual is a dynamic part of a group or environment, with ability to influence and express himself). A teenager might feel that he is subject to the family authority and rules but is not, himself, influential. With friends on the street he may feel more connected as an active contributing member of a coalition or alliance. No matter what his parents think of this connection, it builds self-identity and serves an adaptive purpose for the teenager.

### Connectedness, sense of control, and resistance to depression

If an adolescent's self-identity is based on passive connections, a belief in their ability to effect change in the world is likely to be weak. Eventually, when an event such as failing an exam comes about, the individual may demonstrate a sense of helplessness. "I studied" or "It's not my fault" attributions are likely to be external ("the teacher is unfair – everyone else failed too") and there may be a sense of not being able to make a difference and catastrophic thinking ("I did all I could. I can't do anything else. I'll never be a good student, I might as well drop out").

On the other side of the coin, in relationships where the adolescent is more actively connected, engaged in a cooperative partnership and experiencing a sense of control, there are decreased conditions for depression. Responses to negative situations are likely to reflect a sense of control and ability to move toward a better outcome. "I can't understand it, I studied so hard. There must be a problem, I could talk to the teacher…find out where I went wrong."

#### SCHOOL CONNECTEDNESS

School connectedness predicts academic achievement. Academic achievement is associated more with motivation and resilience than intelligence. In a circular process, motivation and resilience are likely to increase with success in achieving goals. Positive Psychology has identified that challenging activities will result in increased resilience. The experience of connectedness would be a motivating factor to engage in challenging activities in the first place.

Developing school connectedness might include taking part in school activities, taking an active role in the school newspaper or volunteer activities, organization of social events, forming study groups, and taking opportunities to socialize. Personal skills can be utilized to help the school or other students, or in bringing people together with a common goal.

#### FAMILY CONNECTEDNESS

Family connectedness predicts psychological well-being. Positive self-concept and ego development are more likely when parents act in ways that support and challenge autonomy while expressing the importance of family. Examples are in opportunities to express independence; engagement, interaction, and self-disclosure between parents and adolescents; and tolerance of undesired opinions and emotions. In contrast, emotional detachment from parents can be harmful to psychological development.

## SOCIAL AND PEER CONNECTEDNESS

Social and peer connectedness offer opportunities to develop identity within the context of groups including friendships, peers, co-workers, gangs, and sports. For the adolescent, identification with a reference group is often a transitory stage with formative influence. The adolescent is likely to adopt group goals when less mature and form his own relatively stable goals and values later in adolescence and in early adulthood.

## CULTURAL CONNECTEDNESS

Cultural connectedness is demonstrated clearly in a multicultural society. Immigrant adolescents commonly experience being uprooted from their history, language difficulties, alienation, and loss of familiar cultural norms and roles. In response, ethnic minorities are likely to reinforce their cultural identities in order to distinguish themselves from other Americans. Some may "advertise" their differences through maintaining connections with others of the same culture, distinctive clothing, or symbols on their car. Affirming ethnic identity is a strategy that makes connections and strengthens the individual's cultural identity. It is yet another way for the individual to make a place for himself in the larger society.

## CONNECTEDNESS AND SPIRITUALITY OR RELIGION

People who have a personal, emotionally expressive connectedness in church activities are significantly healthier (physically and psychologically) than those who go to church but are not emotionally connected or expressive. In one study, comparing the effect of religious beliefs and behavior in black churches, it was found that attendance of religious services without involvement had little impact on health, yet there was a significant association between good health and involvement with religious crusades, singing, and taking an active part in church activities and organizations (Murray 2000). The distinction between these activities appeared to be participation in emotional self-expression and genuine connectedness.

## Summary: being happy and resilient

Positive emotions are useful building blocks for physical and mental well-being. Being happy lessens the effect of negative events and also enhances potential for new learning and positive change. People can be made happy through easily found pleasures such as jokes, music, and movies. A less emotional but more resilient gratification can result from involvement in activities for which there is a passion or abiding interest – activities which involve meeting a challenge, a sense of accomplishment, making progress in a larger goal or purpose. Emotionally expressive connectedness not only increases resilience and psychological well-being, but also benefits physical health.

The next section of this chapter addresses how we can help adolescents build a foundation with these objectives in mind, the importance of signature strengths, goals, and cognitive and behavioral strategies.

## Helping adolescents get happy

Seligman (2002) argued that happiness throughout life is determined primarily by three things:

- inherited and genetically influenced potential for experiencing happiness – "set range"

- circumstances

- voluntary control.

### Inherited and genetically influenced potential for experiencing happiness – "set range"

Over recent decades much research has been done through twin studies. Twins separated at birth and brought up separately have been studied as adults, comparing the degree of similarities and differences to the similarities and differences that could be expected between two unrelated adults. The results illustrate that a great deal of who we are is inherent. Not only is there an innate tendency to be happy but inherited traits such as introversion/extraversion or optimism/pessimism will have an enormous impact on the interpretation of experience and choices made that could lead to happy experiences.

## Circumstances

A certain level of security is required before happiness can be achieved. Above that threshold, however, there is a weak relationship between wealth and happiness. As mentioned earlier in the introduction to Positive Psychology, research has found that although events, health, and material wealth have some immediate association with happiness, pre-event levels of happiness are likely to return after a time of adaptation.

## Voluntary control

This is essentially the desire and determination to be happy. It is an area where parents and professionals can offer a great deal of therapeutic support. There is little that we can do to change the set range and inherited potential to be happy. Life events will vary according to individual circumstances and we cannot predict or prevent many of them. Voluntary control is the will to control, change, or modify our behavior and reactions to what happens to us. Empowering an individual to have the desire and determination to be happy requires helping them build confidence and skills to be effective in their own environment, effective in making positive choices, and determining the course of their own lives. It requires awareness of the emotion that motivates (or diffuses) effort to take control and that may bias responses to life's events. Parents and professionals can help the adolescent:

- to be more self-conscious about their ability to effect changes
- to make conscious choices in reaction to experiences
- to develop emotions and perceptions that will be empowering (or inhibiting) in making positive choices
- to build skills that will promote a positive response to life events, expected and unexpected
- to develop coping strategies
- to set and achieve short-term and long-term goals
- to anticipate weaknesses in a plan
- to modify "what comes naturally"
- to make links which bring together energy, will, and goals.

Success in treatment or support programs is less attributable to particular techniques and more attributable to the underlying principle of building strengths and instilling of hope for an individual (Seligman 2002). The ultimate objective of support is to empower the individual through building awareness, steps to make changes, and skills to do so.

Big changes start with small steps. Developing a sense of self and control is not likely to come through an intellectual "a-ha" experience in a conversation with a parent or therapist. It is more likely to develop through practice, small but significant successes, awareness and appreciation of personal strengths, and development of tools from visualization of a concept to completion of a goal.

The first step is to identify strengths that are intrinsic to the adolescent and will support him in his goals and endeavors. The kind of personal strengths that are instrumental in constructing and experiencing a fulfilled life include the 24 personal strengths identified by Seligman in *Authentic Happiness* (2002):

- curiosity/interest in the world
- love of learning
- judgment/critical thinking/open-mindedness
- ingenuity/originality/practical intelligence/street smarts
- social intelligence/personal intelligence/emotional intelligence
- perspective
- valor and bravery
- perseverance/industry/diligence
- integrity/genuineness/honesty
- kindness and generosity
- loving and allowing oneself to be loved
- citizenship/duty/teamwork/loyalty
- fairness and equity
- leadership
- self-control
- prudence/discretion/caution
- humility and modesty
- appreciation of beauty and excellence
- gratitude

- hope/optimism/future-mindedness
- spirituality/sense of purpose/faith/religiousness
- forgiveness and mercy
- playfulness and humor
- zest/passion/enthusiasm.

A website that more comprehensively explains the 24 strengths can be found at http://www.authentichappiness.org/strengths.html, developed by Christopher Peterson and Martin Seligman (2004). It is reproduced with permission in Appendix 1. Seligman recommends that more effort is put into identification and development of stronger "signature" strengths than focusing on areas where there is little interest or natural inclination.

> Identification of five strengths which are dominant in a personality gives a key to innate characteristics that will offer resilience in the face of depression and negative life events, and will help in choosing appropriate goals and finding strategies to achieve them.

The wish for succeess and positive goals is not enough. Motivation and personal skills are needed to complete them. Csikszentmihalyi (1997) writes: "Emotions focus attention by mobilizing the entire organism in an approach or an avoidance mode; goals do it by providing images of desired outcomes." Emotions and goals work together to harness motivation (energy) and direction. The emotional component provides energy (or lack of energy).

Just as practicing driving a car will eventually result in skills becoming almost automatic, social and emotional skills are most effective when they have been practiced to a degree of fluency. Jonathan Cohen (2001) refers to the importance of "literacy" in social and emotional skills and argues that it is just as important as any other language or intelligence in negotiation through the world.

We turn to the model of Social and Emotional Learning. While overlapping with principles of Positive Psychology, SEL focuses on "principles of internal development" (Cohen 2001) that enhance learning and development.

## Social and Emotional Learning (SEL)

The Positive Psychology and SEL models complement each other, both affirming the need to identify and use strengths, consider values, responsibility, and a genuine connection with others in positive development. In the model of Positive Psychology, Seligman uses signature strengths to construct a fulfilled and positive life. Csikszentmihalyi uses strengths to engage in meaningful activities, and meaningful activities contribute to a gratified and positive life.

The SEL model focuses on the social and emotional skills that support positive life goals, and the need to have social and emotional skills in order to access and develop values, responsibility, and genuine connection. Social and emotional skills provide a language of negotiation. All of these factors combine, overlap, and complement each other in supporting the individual toward a conscious, skilled, responsible autonomy.

Social and emotional competence has been defined as the ability to understand, process, manage, and express the social and emotional aspects of our lives. The degree to which we are able to do so is predictive of life satisfaction and productivity (Cohen 2001).

*If life is to be lived to its potential, it cannot afford to be lived by default*

Habit, a limited perspective, or inability to understand alternative ways of thinking and behaving will make our lives and well-being very vulnerable to events over which we have little control. We might want positive changes but not have the ability to effect change. We will be carried along by the conditions that come into our lives, with an inability to make much significant difference – riding in the back seat of the car rather than driving.

On the other hand, with realistic awareness of ourselves and skills to overcome self-imposed boundaries, more options are possible. Life can be approached with an inquiring mind, guided by ideals. Opportunities to communicate, learn, adapt, and interact with self-respect and responsibility will enlarge potential. Social and emotional skills ideally enhance autonomy and cooperation, purpose and resilience. Social and emotional skills support personal control and effective negotiation with the environment.

*Principles and ideals of social and emotional skills*

Why do some individuals have more social and emotional "fluency" than others? Are these skills innate? We do not know the degree to which they are innate but they can certainly be modified. Ability to develop useful social and emotional skills in young children rests largely on the following principles identified by Mugno and Rosenblitt (2001). These principles are also relevant to adolescent development:

- subjective perspectives
- meaningfulness of behavior
- adaptation
- relationships
- fluidity
- delay and deviation
- conflict.

## SUBJECTIVE PERSPECTIVES

Subjective perspectives are the biases that each individual has. It is unrealistic to expect to be free of bias, individual thoughts, beliefs, and fears. It is helpful to be aware of individual perspectives and biases. A fundamental social emotional skill is the awareness of bias, and ability for the individual to stand back from their own experience and see alternative perspectives.

## MEANINGFULNESS OF BEHAVIOR

This relates to underlying reasons, which sometimes might be clear. (A teenage girl's argument with parents about staying out late may be because she feels they are being unreasonable.) There may be other less obvious reasons. (She is angry because she believes every aspect of her life is controlled or she feels she is not trusted.) A basic social emotional skill is awareness of underlying meanings for behavior.

## ADAPTATION, FLUIDITY, DELAY, AND DEVIATION

These are all relevant to adolescence. Life appeared to be fairly simple when there were concrete ways of looking at things, Mom and Dad made the most important decisions, and there was little need for long-term goals and compromise. Adolescence brings with it a need to integrate new information, new ways of processing it, changes that come with transitions. Not all adolescents have the maturity and resources to meet those demands on the same level.

Losses and transitions include changes of schools and friends. New ways of learning are expected at high school and college level. Writing evaluative essays rather than reporting learned facts is not a smooth transition for some teenagers – especially for the child who had excelled because of an innate talent for memorizing facts. There is an increased expectation of independence such as ability to design a study plan without supervision. Friendships have different rules and are more complex than in younger years. An adolescent girl is expected to deal appropriately with the attention her body is suddenly attracting.

Reactions to transitions might be expressed in unexpected or destructive ways. The freedom that comes with increasing independence might be abused through late nights or disregard for family rules, drinking alcohol, or experimenting with drugs. The sudden interest by the opposite gender may result in undesirable behavior. Some adolescents may withdraw into themselves or find uncharacteristic ways to express their dissatisfaction with the world. Social emotional skills to handle experiences of adaptation, delay, and deviation will facilitate transitions of adolescence.

RELATIONSHIPS

Relationships can provide supportive associations yet strengthen conditions for autonomy. Adolescents benefit from significant relationships with caring others. Genuine connectedness with others provides an anchor, offering some stability in a time of emotional instability. Relationships may be particularly volatile in teen years, in keeping with other dynamics of adolescence. Yet, as discussed earlier, the most beneficial relationships are reciprocal. The quality of the relationships will depend largely on what the individual brings to them. Self-awareness, consciousness, and deliberate behavior are required for self-responsibility. It is helpful to clarify what the adolescent can contribute to his or her relationships in order to make and maintain healthy connections.

CONFLICT

Conflict relates to the inner defenses and self-protective strategies that have developed but may interfere with positive choices and behavior. Emotional dilemmas motivate and inhibit behavior. As in previous principles, increased awareness of self is fundamental to developing the appropriate social and emotional skills. It is only with awareness of the role played by one's own emotions, perspectives, values, and sense of responsibility that cognitive and behavioral changes can be deliberate.

*How can we develop those principles and idealistic skills in the individuals with whom we work?*

These principles can be integrated into behavior through self-awareness and consciousness. With skills of awareness and consciousness, we do not live "accidentally" but are able to identify, adapt, manage, resolve, and learn new ways of thinking and behaviors. More specifically, modification and development of social and emotional competencies and skills will relate to the following categories:

- *self-awareness* (awareness of self and own emotions, ability to "decode," understand and label emotions, self-regulation, communication, self-motivation, realistic and positive sense of self)

- *social awareness and interaction* (awareness of others, ability to "decode," understand and respect their perspective, appreciating the differences of others, collaboration)

- *self-management*, responsible and purposeful behavior (problem solving, decision making, realistic analysis, ability to set and work toward goals).

The emotional component of skills is important because "emotional life influences and often determines behavior…we do not always recognize what we feel; learning how to read emotions – our own and others" (Cohen 2001). We are responsible for the choices we make. Awareness of emotions and employment of skills plays a crucial role in the ability to make positive and responsible choices. Some of the emotional and social skills, such as perspective and self-control, overlap with strengths central to development in Positive Psychology. Parents and professionals can integrate both models for cues to build valuable competencies and strengths.

A pattern emerges from the information in this section. Similar principles are fundamental to both models although they may be categorized or worded differently. Familiarity with the concepts is invaluable because they can then be integrated in different ways, informally as well as formally, in programs, in conversations, in interactions at school and home. The SEL model is designed to function primarily in an educational setting; the Positive Psychology model relates well to personal development and therapy. However, the principles complement and reinforce each other. Continuing with the SEL model, we have identified:

- principles (such as being able to delay gratification, overcome biases, interact with others) that provide the goals for building social and emotional skills

- that to reach those ideals and goals, the individual must be self-aware, self-conscious in behavior, and responsible for himself.

Self-awareness, self-consciousness, and self-responsibility rarely just happen and cannot be imposed. The individual must be engaged in the idea that they are active participants in their world and what unfolds around them. This is the essence of responsible maturity. It can be a very exciting process of realization and empowerment.


## Engaging in self-awareness, consciousness, and responsibility

Cohen (2001) has identified five concepts that are central to building emotional and social skills in young children. They are tools to support development of self-awareness and responsibility and can be used effectively with adolescents:

- reflectiveness
- problem solving
- safe responsive environments
- school–home–community collaboration
- creative learning.


### Reflectiveness

For Cohen (2001), reflectiveness is a "process of discovery about emotional truths or knowledge". It increases awareness of values, thoughts and feelings, attitudes, desires, and fears. It is not only directed internally. Reflectiveness encourages observational and listening skills, opening doors for new information from other people. It allows us to "decode" our own behavior and the behavior of others – to recognize patterns, possible motivations, and ways of communication. Self-reflection can be used to identify goals that are important to the individual and for which there is intrinsic motivation. Reflectiveness can identify strengths to support goals and possible obstacles.

Reflectiveness facilitates a realistic self-awareness. High self-esteem empowers people to make positive choices. But development of high self-esteem does not evolve from being told "You're very special" or having success come too easily. High self-esteem may cause more trouble than good if it is not grounded in reality. Consequently, it is useful to recall and build on small achievements, and direct energy into goals which would build and support a realistic, positive sense of self.

Self-esteem and self-concept make distinct contributions to positive development. Self-concept is how the individual identifies himself ("I am a tennis player; I am a student"). Self-esteem is evaluative ("I am a good tennis player; I am a poor student"). Without reflectiveness or consciousness, an adolescent may have a simple self-concept of just a couple of aspects (student, son). Life may seem to revolve around these few domains and when failure or disappointment are experienced, there is little resilience. If the adolescent fails his exams and feels he has disappointed his parents, the effect could be devastating.

However, if the adolescent has a more complex self-concept (student, son, debate team member, class clown, friend, guitar player, CD collector, inventor, would-be lawyer) more parts of his identity can act as a safety net to support his sense of self if failure is experienced in one or two areas. Rowitz and Jurkowski (1995) have studied the effect of leisure activities on people with significant mental health issues. They found that 75 percent of people with no leisure activities had very high depression, compared to 9.59 percent of those involved with more than seven activities.

A worthwhile goal of support for the adolescent is to find ways to increase complexity of self-concept. Reflectiveness may increase awareness of multiple aspects of self and lead to developing more aspects of self.

## Problem solving

Problem solving is related to language skills, ability to observe, listen, communicate, and cooperate. Useful skills include the ability to analyze and break down a problem, see different perspectives or the problem as a whole rather than partially, make links and be creative in discovering possible solutions, and the ability to set relevant short-term and long-term goals. The purposeful behavior involved in problem solving also requires attention, the ability to concentrate and pursue an objective, foreseeing and overcoming obstacles. Skills in this area may perceive a problem as a challenge to be met, with implications for motivation and tenacity in resolution.

## Safe responsive environments

Safe responsive environments provide conditions that will nurture the individual and their development of social and emotional skills. While this is most important for a young child who has little autonomy, it is also very relevant to the adolescent who is taking tentative steps toward independence. It is in this world of half child–half adult that significant relationships are very important, encouraging autonomy in the context of a responsive and supportive connectedness. This relates a great deal to the fourth concept of ideal conditions for development of social and environmental skills – significant connections and relationships to other people.

## School–home–community collaboration

School–home–community collaboration requires interaction and cooperation between different environmental domains. School–home–community collaboration is also very similar to the concept that is referred to with connectedness that has proven to be beneficial for mental and physical health. When the individual feels he has a reciprocal relationship with home, school, and community, and there is an integration of those relationships, there are opportunities for authentic growth in self-consciousness and responsibility. This is an area where professionals and parents can work together to identify and encourage potential collaborative and reciprocal relationships in the adolescent's life.

## Creative learning

Finally, creative learning is one of the five concepts introduced by Cohen as useful for building social and emotional skills. In turn, social and emotional skills enhance creative learning. This concept is close to the heart of this book. Creativity expands self-consciousness through opportunities to realize, acknowledge, and express the individual's unique perspective.

No two paintings will be the same, even with the same materials. Similarly, no two lives will be the same, even under similar circumstances. Many artists will strive to paint like someone else, or focus on technical sophistication at the expense of genuine self-expression. Many adolescents will strive to dress like others, copy a lifestyle, be seen to be sophisticated. Yet nobody can ever truly assume someone else's identity, style or life – it's a set-up for failure. The value of creativity is the unique contribution that each individual brings to the choices he makes. Being given permission and skills to respond to life with our own authentic and creative response offers resilience in itself. Positive outcomes due to self-conscious and responsible choices will add to the resilience.

Creativity can be integrated into different activities during everyday life, used to generate novel responses to a dilemma or problem. Creative responses to life open alternative and often more positive ways of living, congruent with the goal of increased consciousness and breaking down habitual ways of thinking. The nature of creativity is that it requires choices to be made, employing and developing social and emotional competencies along the way.

Creativity enhances behavior and life through increased self-consciousness. What is your experience with peaches? Do you remember when you last ate a peach? Where were you? What did it taste like? Unless it was very recently, or a novel experience in an unusual place or circumstances, you probably don't remember. Yet, eat a peach "creatively" and see how the effort changes the experience. Push your creativity by eating a peach in a different way, every day for a year – combine your peach with other foods, invent a new tool to stone it, use it in novel ways. Creative solutions open up new worlds. Creativity draws on resources unique and available to each individual. It provides an expressive, rich network and means to actualize thoughts, feelings, skills, strengths, potential, ideas, and ideals. Creative expression is literally limited only by the imagination.

In informal, everyday, and elemental ways, creativity has a generative relationship with social and emotional skills. It encourages and rewards curiosity, problem solving, goal setting, intrinsic motivation and tenacity, novel perceptions and interpretations. It is contingent upon uniqueness and different perspectives. Working creatively with others opens a new world of possibilities in cooperation, negotiation, and team building.

Creativity in response to life events makes a strong contribution to a positive and fulfilling life. It takes more effort than living in "remote control" and it is unrealistic to be creative all the time in every situation. But creative thinking becomes easier with practice and, when used, a creative approach and response will give more control and more reward over life events. Creative activities have many of the characteristics identified by Csikszenmihalyi (1996) in the experience of flow: "When we are involved in it, we feel that we are living more fully than during the rest of life."

With the principles of Positive Psychology and the supporting Social and Emotional Learning models in mind, how does Asperger's Syndrome impact on healthy and resilient development?

# CHAPTER 3

# Defining Asperger's Syndrome and its impact

What this life will amount to is in part determined by the chemical processes in our body, by the biological interaction among organs, by the tiny electrical currents jumping between the synapses of the brain, and by the organization of information that the culture imposes on our mind. But the actual quality of life – what we do, and how we feel about it – will be determined by our thoughts and emotions; by the interpretations we give to chemical, biological and social processes. (Mihaly Csikszentmihalyi)

## Introduction to Asperger's Syndrome

Asperger's Syndrome was identified as a pattern of traits about 50 years ago by Hans Asperger. Knowledge about it has expanded considerably since then, particularly in the last ten years. The complexity of the syndrome is still emerging and there are mixed theories but no conclusion about its cause. Sometimes Asperger's Syndrome is easily identified. Obsessive behavior, literal speech, or intolerance of some sensory stimulation typically signpost the AS pattern. Sometimes, however, behaviors are not strong enough to be diagnosed as part of the Asperger pattern and are seen as simply quirky or eccentric personality traits.

For those with very strong traits of Asperger's, there may be difficulties in adulthood with independent living, employment, and relationships. Yet for others, traits such as differences in thought processing may be more subtle and individuals seen simply as unconventional, eccentric, or difficult. As they get older, many people will learn through experience and observation, developing skills and modifying their behavior accordingly.

Individuals with mild Asperger traits are very capable of living fulfilled and independent lives, never identified as having Asperger's Syndrome. Universities are familiar with the eccentric academic who is obsessed with his science yet has little time for people, absorbed, highly skilled, and thorough in his work, content to work in relative isolation, typically not socially motivated or professionally ambitious.

Asperger's Syndrome is a classification for a group of characteristics and traits common to the autistic spectrum. Sometimes Asperger's Syndrome is called high-functioning autism, although AS does not share all the autistic traits. For example, there are cognitive delays in the development of autistic children but generally not with AS; there is often a clumsiness and motor disorders such as Tourette's Disorder concurrent with AS that is not evident in autism; a desire for friendship and social interaction typically in AS people that is not shared by autistic people; and generally a higher intelligence level in AS individuals although that may be related to better communication skills. The DSM-IV-TR (American Psychiatric Association 2000) specifies in detail the criteria for a diagnosis of Asperger's Syndrome. Broadly, they include:

- at least two examples of impairment of social interaction which might be demonstrated through nonverbal behaviors, difficulties in maintaining relationships with peers, reluctance to initiate sharing activities with other people, or limited social and emotional interaction

- repetitive behavior or exaggerated interest in particular activities or objects

- characteristic traits so strong that they are causing problems in the individual's ability to function in their environment

- no significant developmental delay in language, cognitive development, or other behavior typical of a child of the same young age (as there would be for a diagnosis of autism).

Two observations can be made immediately from these criteria. First, AS traits predominantly demonstrate weaknesses in social and emotional skills, which provide building blocks for healthy and positive development, the topic of Part I of this book. The exaggerated interests (or obsessions) are a distinctive trait, but unless they cause dysfunction in life they are not the central issue. (If repetitive, obsessive behavior is causing dysfunction, a secondary diagnosis and treatment for Obsessive Compulsive Disorder may be appropriate.) The most obvious need for support of individuals with Asperger's Syndrome is in the area of social and emotional skills.

Second, the DSM list of criteria does not offer a clear road map for treatment and support. It does not list many of the characteristics common to Asperger's Syndrome such as the literal, concrete thinking and the difficulty in seeing other people's perspective. Parents and professionals may benefit from using diagnosis as a cue to explain associated characteristics that sometimes (not always) occur with AS, such as a tendency toward mood disorders, depression or hypomania, Tourette's Disorder, sleep difficulties, and inexplicable emotional outbursts such as crying and aggression.

In a group of people with Asperger's Syndrome, the strong and unique individuality of each member will give the impression that they have little in common. Nevertheless, the traits commonly (although not always) experienced include the following:

1. Difficulties and complications with or shortly after birth, such as forceps delivery, and possible delay in speech development but, generally, normal early development.

2. Generally a pleasant temperament and lack of deceit or malice; a keen sense of fairness and dislike of injustice to self and others; a sense of honesty that can give offense when expressed without diplomacy and typical lack of tact; generally cooperative; a naivety that can lead to victimization.

3. Lack of understanding of their own and others' emotions; difficulty in acting out complex emotions such as sadness; inappropriate or limited range of facial expressions and difficulty in distinguishing between facial expressions in other people; difficulties with facial recognition of other people; discomfort with maintaining eye contact with others, or a tendency to stare inappropriately or have a peculiar gaze.

4. Pedantic, literal speech and interpretation; precise enunciation; mechanical tone or flat affect in voice, or unusual inflection, pronunciation, or speed; difficulties in articulating thoughts; tendency to interrupt others, to either speak too much or be withdrawn, preoccupied with their own thoughts; reluctance to admit they are wrong about something, or take responsibility for something that has gone wrong; problems with initiating and maintaining a conversation appropriately.

5. Difficulties in understanding humor or finding humor in jokes not appreciated by other people; inappropriate laughter; inappropriate

sense of space, standing either too close or too far from people; an assumption that other people know what he or she is thinking and even share the same thoughts and feelings; unable to understand why parents worry about his or her behavior.

6. Clumsiness, unbalanced or poor gross motor skills (causing a dislike of ball games), and poor fine motor skills (untidy handwriting); typically a lack of competitiveness and inability to see the point of team sports and ball games; an unusual or heavy gait.

7. Peculiar, repetitive movement of part of the body or facial grimaces; sensitivity to color, taste, or texture of food; acutely sensitive to light (particularly fluorescent flickering), smells, temperature, touch (seams of socks, labels of clothes); overly sensitive or impervious to pain.

8. Intense, special interest (or obsession) with some objects or subjects; accumulation of things and information for themselves rather than their function; excellent memory for details and facts, although often unable to relate them to a larger picture or understand implicit meaning; memory is often stored visually and cannot be adapted in novel or generalized ways (e.g. recalling the idea of a "vacation" will bring to mind a specific holiday that has been experienced rather than the concept of a vacation).

9. Rigidity in behavior, inability to make transitions well, or accept changes or spontaneous behavior of others; a desire for familiarity including routines and rules, and distress when routines and rules are broken; attraction to ritual or repetition even when it serves no function.

10. Lack of importance may be given to norms such as personal hygiene; unusual or eccentric dress and appearance; poor muscle tone; may be seen as geeks or nerds by peers because of peculiarities; the center of their own world, happy in their self-centeredness with little need for interaction with other people; can prefer solitude.

11. Desire to make friends but difficulty in doing so; lack of understanding what's expected and wanted by others in friendship; apparent lack of empathy or interest in others (out of sight, out of mind); lacking social rules of reciprocity or give and take; will dominate a conversation with monologues, inappropriate topics, and

lack of awareness that he is boring others; may want to control games or social situations and have difficulty taking turns; impulsiveness, frustration, irritability, tendency to thoughtlessly hurt self or others; lack of emotional reciprocity, difficulties in building relationships with same age peers particularly after entering teenage years; a liking for smaller children or older people with whom they may feel more of an affinity (children are more concrete, less demanding; older people more appreciative of their individuality); problems with intimate relationships may arise from literal interpretation, lack of self-knowledge, lack of interest or knowledge of others in relationships, poor intuition, missing behavioral cues and subtleties in others, difficulties with compromise and ability to see the bigger picture or solve problems.

12. Easily distracted, often through sensory sensitivity (noise, lights, surroundings, clothes) or internal pictures and dialogue (resulting from associative thought); higher than average tendency toward conditions such as gastrointestinal problems, sleep problems, obsessive compulsiveness, seizures, bipolar depression.

13. Concrete thinking and lack of hypothetical thought, difficulties in making connections between experience, ideas, concepts, and reasons; inability to give meaning to experience, better at rote learning; lack of ability to pick up on implication or hidden meanings; living in the moment rather than goal-oriented behavior; a desire to be organized (familiarity of orderliness) can be undermined by difficulties in planning and sequencing, due mainly to inability to see the "whole picture" and work toward it consistently and appropriately; difficulties with budgeting and organizing money; reluctance to start something unless it can be done perfectly; dislike of being seen to fail or thought stupid; weaknesses in self-regulation (although will adhere to rules); tendency to think out loud; tendency to use visual aids for learning and recall.

14. Anxiety, cognitive tiredness, and frustration together with inability to identify and handle emotions appropriately, sometimes resulting in outbursts of aggression. These outbursts are typically a release of emotion rather than with a direction or purpose. Greater risk of suicide, possibly triggered by depression, experience of rejection, or

sense of isolation. There may be a tendency to use alcohol, some drugs, or food to self-medicate and ease the anxiety and negative emotions.

As mentioned earlier, there is a range in ability to adapt to the environment. Many AS traits are going to be evident in people who are functioning very well in their environments. Most individuals with Asperger's Syndrome will have at least one other member in their family who can identify with some of the same traits, perhaps to a lesser degree. Relatives may not experience the degree of problem in functioning that is necessary for a diagnosis but could still benefit from strengthening social and emotional skills.

Because AS is a pervasive developmental disorder (or innate wiring of the brain), therapeutic goals toward being "normal" will set up conditions for frustration and failure. Instead, goals should be to modify behavior and skills to adapt to the environment. Skills can be seen as a form of language and the more fluent the individual becomes with them, the easier adaptation will be. As with any language, they should be practiced in a variety of ways and over a period of time.

Conventional programs for children and adolescents with Asperger's Syndrome consist predominantly of cognitive and behavioral exercises to develop language, play, and social skills. Familiarity comes with practice, which in turn generalizes more easily to the schoolyard, classroom, home, and other settings. It must be remembered too that individuals with Asperger's Syndrome have some remarkable strengths which can be used to their advantage. Drawing on signature strengths is a central path to a lifetime of fulfillment.

It is important that adolescents are partners in identifying their needs and the benefits in modifying their behavior. They are likely to complain that they have learned and done it all before. Indeed, they may have an intellectual knowledge of social skills. Multimodal techniques bring a different perspective to practice of skills and reinforce their development. For example, an individual might "know" that he should maintain eye contact and have an understanding of appropriate body language and personal space while maintaining a conversation. A videotape of a role play might be an effective tool for its visual impact.

There are three areas that are typical of Asperger's Syndrome and therefore likely to impact on the principles of positive development discussed in Chapter 2:

- conceptual and cognitive processing: semantic and pragmatic weaknesses

- self-awareness and self-related skills: emotion, depression, anxiety, emotional self-regulation

- social difficulties and connecting with the world beyond self.

## Conceptual and cognitive processing

*Semantic and pragmatic weaknesses: lack of integration between mind and body*

There is individuality within Asperger's Syndrome and not all people have the same traits. However, a characteristic of AS is non-conventional ways of perceiving, thinking, and retrieving memories. Some of these can be used to advantage, such as an eye and memory for minute visual details, or an almost photographic memory. Some differences make interaction with the rest of the world difficult. In addition there is typically a lack of integration or co-ordination between the mind and body which impacts on complex learning and living tasks.

Unfortunately many individuals with AS feel stupid as well as different. On one level, they know they are not stupid, yet they manage to mess up things that other people find very easy. A fundamental problem is the interruption in the process of receiving, organizing, integrating, and expressing information that enables intelligence to be realized. This is comparable to someone designing and building a unique and beautiful boat in their backyard but not knowing who or how to ask for help to transport it to the ocean. It can be done but is so much more hard work for the AS individual to get it all together. It also means that many valuable ideas will never have their potential fulfilled.

SENSORY INTEGRATION

The difficulty in integration and processing of simple sensory tasks is manifested in different ways and in different levels of severity. It may be in the form of dyspraxia, apraxia, Developmental Co-ordination Disorder, clumsiness, motor learning difficulties, or auditory processing difficulties. Often, exposure and experience through specific activities is the best teacher. (For example, touching non-responsive parts of the mouth may act to increase sensitivity and responsiveness in those areas and help articulation.)

This book takes a broad approach, with suggestions for support activities for a range of typical traits. It serves as an introduction to an integrated and comprehensive support, rather than focusing on one area at the expense of others. For more intense support in an area, specialized professionals such as speech therapists, occupational therapists, or audiologists should be consulted.

Positive, adaptive, and resilient development depends largely on the ability to integrate the five senses, along with the sense of body awareness and movement. This integration typically causes difficulty for people with Asperger's Syndrome. They tend to be either overly or under-sensitive in some or all of the senses. For most of us, sensory information is a yardstick to start, stop, or change direction. For the AS individual, such information is distorted or not integrated appropriately.

Sensory awareness and integration is an area where creative activities – combining skills and senses in novel exercises – can be very helpful. Objectives and goals should include experience, integration, modification, and regulation of music, color, taste, light, texture, movement, two- and three-dimensional art, and so on. Recognizing areas of weakness facilitates introduction of experiences in casual and informal contexts. For example, helping in the kitchen creating a recipe will call for integration of taste (does it taste right?), color (does it look overcooked?), tactile experiences (is it too dry?), motor skills, and planning and sequencing skills.

In Part II of this book, there are some activities that are designed to address sensory integration and dyspraxia together. Dyspraxia describes weaknesses such as co-ordination of gross motor skills (dancing, movement) and fine motor skills (writing, craft work), combining tasks, controlled and economical movement of the body and its different parts (even eyes), a lack of organization in language, speech, memory, time sequencing, picking up and correct perception of environmental cues. Other than the practical consequences that these weaknesses present, there are the emotional repercussions – feeling "stupid," "weird," "not like other people," and frustrated.

ABSTRACT THINKING

An AS adolescent typically has some difficulties with hypothetical and abstract thinking. Without AS, thinking processes usually become less concrete and more abstract from the ages of 12 or 13. Problem solving relies less on "rules" and more on hypothetical reasoning. The teenager is increasingly able to predict a specific outcome based on general principles. Relative thinking is used, shades of gray are allowed in arguments, and perspective is seen to be subjective. At the same time, methods of teaching and testing in school change. Learned facts, an area where the AS individual often excels, become less important. Educators encourage consideration of many sides to a question rather than requiring one "right" answer. Testing includes assignments that require independent thinking about a subject, supported by arguments that extend beyond simple recall of learned information.

Adolescents with Asperger traits typically remain more concrete and literal than their non-AS peers, demonstrating little imagination beyond their own experience. Writing essays based on opinions or reactions, with no right or wrong answers, can be confusing. Many AS individuals see the world from their egocentric perspective and have difficulty understanding the world from perspectives they have not experienced. They may be experts in specific topics, able to list facts about a subject in which they have an interest, but intelligence also requires flexibility of thinking and interpretation of information. AS adolescents tend to be less comfortable in these areas. Asking about a movie they have seen will typically result in a detailed description, scene by scene, without a conceptual idea of the movie or discussion of meaning. The best way to counter this is exposure and awareness of a variety of opinions and perspectives – often a byproduct of maturity, time, traveling, and mixing and working with other people.

A very important implication for concrete thinking and literal interpretation is the effect it is likely to have on personal relationships. During the adolescent years, the AS individual will need to learn new ways of building friendships and close relationships. They may expect to date and perhaps marry. The rules of childhood – with concrete thinking – no longer work. Literal interpretation of what another person says, particularly in arguments, can have unfortunate consequences. Learning how to compromise and negotiate in relationships is necessary for maturity and resilience.

SYMBOLIC THOUGHT

The limited ability to make inferences from personal experience demonstrates a lack of symbolic thought and has implications for problem solving and achieving goals. Normally, symbolic thought is acquired along with language. Through pretend play with objects and people, the young child learns that toys and words are symbols for real things and ideas. Following that is a slow realization that things can be categorized.

For a two-year-old a car is the big machine that takes the family to the shop. After some time and exposure, broader and general assumptions can be made about them (they all have wheels) but differentiation and comparisons can be made too (types, colors, sizes). Eventually, given interest and knowledge of the principles that make up a "car," an individual can invent a new and unique type of car. The inventor will probably use both verbal and visual symbols (words and pictures) to communicate his idea of this unique car to other people, so that they can "see" it, even though such a car is still just an idea, not real. As the idea becomes clear, progress can be made toward making it a reality.

We constantly deal in ideas and concepts – planning for a party or a future, anticipating difficulties with school, work, relationships, and possible solutions. Ideas are represented, symbolized, and developed through verbal and visual language. Being able to understand and communicate in ideas and concepts is essential to being adaptive and resilient.

As adults, we become more adept at acquiring a concept and then fitting detailed information into that concept. Temple Grandin (1995) makes the distinction between the non-Asperger individual who can acquire a concept and then fit information to that concept, and the Asperger individual who acquires a concept through repeated experiences of detailed information, gradually forming a picture that integrates what has been experienced.

Being able to categorize information and organize it according to patterns of similarities and differences gives grounds for reasoning. A framework of information with expected outcomes and consequences can be built, into which new or hypothetical information finds a place. These frameworks or schemas are the tools for problem solving and abstract thinking. Conceptual thinking plays a crucial role in the goals, tasks, problem solving, and creative thinking that are important in healthy adolescent development.

For the AS individual, information should ideally be presented in ways that integrate detailed information into a bigger picture, making inferences and drawing implications, prioritizing information, setting goals, and problem solving. At the same time, sentences and questions should be short and simple, without complex grammatical structure, and not using long sequences of ideas, leaving the individual to interpret meaning from those sequences. Verbal and visual languages reinforce each other.

ORGANIZATION

Independence requires ability to set goals, along with the skills necessary to organize completion of them. Organization of information and life in general can cause problems for the AS individual. In order to achieve the simplest goal, there has to be an overall view of the process toward a desired outcome.

Cooking a cake, going to school, driving a car, even getting married, usually involve short- or long-term goals. Sometimes goals are clear, sometimes they are not.

If an AS person has a picture in his head of the finished goal, he is probably able to figure out the process needed to get there. If the goal is not clear, there is likely to be confusion about the required steps and action to be taken. Younger children may have to be shown how to pack a bag or a cupboard because they cannot do it on their own. To make matters worse, being hurried or overwhelmed with frustration can lead to a meltdown. Routine and a checklist will make life at home easier. As the individual gets older and begins work, a checklist of expectations, duties, or chores might be more productive than being left to use initiative on the job. Temple Grandin has some difficulty with the sequences of processes but she remedies this by making visual maps or cues.

The inability to hold more than two or three things in the mind at one time is demonstrated in what appears to be a lack of concentration, difficulty in staying on track in a conversation, or going off at seemingly unrelated tangents. Distraction can also occur easily through sensory reaction to the environment (visual distractions, fluorescent lights, noise, scratchy clothes). The individual may have an accurate awareness of detail but difficulty in relating it and integrating it into a cohesive whole.

As the adolescent moves through school, college, and into the workplace, attention to detail can be useful in some contexts but amount to reinventing the wheel in others. A great deal of assistance can be given with prioritizing and discerning when detail is important and when it is relatively unimportant. Support and guidance can be given in identifying strategies for organization (from study habits to financial planning), using visual charts, timelines, and various ways of reaching goals. As an example, many have a remarkable memory for information that has been stored visually. One university student with AS traits found that a study strategy in writing essays was to lay information out on sheets of paper across the floor, representing a conceptual map of a tree trunk and branches. With this structure, clusters of information could then be retrieved visually according to their position on the "tree" and elaborated upon in the essay.

PRAGMATICS AND SEMANTICS

Weaknesses in the pragmatics and semantics of language – understanding and articulation – are commonly experienced by people on the autistic spectrum.

Some professionals consider it a distinctive characteristic of individuals with autism and Asperger's Syndrome. Every consideration should be made to design therapeutic activities with this in mind – both in design of actual activities, and in their presentation. Pragmatics refers to language used in social interaction. Pragmatic language includes unspoken social rules – knowing how to appropriately contribute to a conversation, what to say, taking turns, appropriate volume, and subject matter – and how to be socially appropriate in social conversation. These implicit rules are considered good manners or basic common sense to most people. Individuals with AS can be socially clumsy unless the rules are spelt out, and even then they may be inadvertently rude or bore new acquaintances with long and uninteresting monologues (such as a 20-minute detailed explanation on the best roads to take to get from A to B). When they are made aware of the social rules and expectations, it can be hard work and stressful to remain conscious of appropriate social interaction. For some, the hard work component may lead to avoidance of social situations.

Semantics is related to word meaning. AS individuals frequently have an admirable knowledge of language and can be quite pedantic about using the correct words. Yet the same characteristic can cause them to become "stuck" on words that cannot be used literally. There may be problems comprehending a sentence with complicated grammatical structure or abstract concepts. The essence of the sentence will be lost and the AS individual will go off at an unrelated tangent – sometimes just in his head so that the teacher or parent is unaware that the point has been missed and the listener is following a completely different track in their mind. Semantic difficulties can cause of a lot of misunderstanding and frustration. They can cause the AS individual to feel stupid or be considered lacking in common sense by others. Parents and teachers may feel their children are careless in listening, being uncooperative or deliberately causing trouble. In reaction to frustrated efforts to understand and be understood and consequent feelings of low self-esteem, the adolescent may withdraw or be prone to meltdowns.

## Self-awareness and self-related skills
*Emotion, depression, anxiety, emotional self-regulation*
The principles of Positive Psychology relate healthy development to skills of perspective, perseverance, loving and allowing one's self to be loved, self-control, gratitude, and playfulness – and the ability to integrate them. Important social and emotional skills include awareness of self, and emotions, ability to understand and label those emotions, motivation, a realistic and positive

sense of self, and reflectiveness. Being authentic to ourselves is a core component to resilience.

With or without traits of Asperger's Syndrome, the way we think and feel about our lives defines the goals we set and motivation to follow through on them. It is ironic that while AS individuals are so self-centered, they can be so unselfconscious. Thus, perhaps the single most useful objective in supporting an adolescent with AS traits is to help increase self-knowledge and consciousness.

## STRENGTHS

Positive adolescent development benefits greatly from building on innate signature strengths and instilling hope. At this point we return to the concept of "flow" activities – those activities which provide a sense of fulfillment. The individual makes an active connection and contribution, meeting challenges, learning, growing, and achieving. Rather than passively having life flow over and around him, he is able to connect and flow with it.

What does AS bring to the picture? Individuals with AS traits have a natural gift for activities that produce flow. One of the most distinctive Asperger traits is obsessions. An obsession is an interest taken to an extreme. Reframing an "obsession" as a "passionate interest" may turn it around to be a positive and manageable first step toward productive, goal-oriented activities that build potential and provide fulfillment. In fact, being obsessive about a subject can result in becoming uncommonly knowledgeable about it.

Modifying Csikszentmihalyi's methods of research to measure happiness, a journal can be used to record the feelings and thoughts associated with different daily experiences. It is possible to identify patterns of interest, motivation, and satisfaction. It is also helpful to identify areas associated with discomfort (such as socially demanding situations), areas where the individual enjoys spending a great deal of time (on the computer), or times when mood can be affected by physical factors (hunger, noise). Identifying patterns of weakness and strength is the key to effective modification, for both immediate and future situations.

## SELF-REGULATION

Disappointment and frustration are inevitable in life. Self-regulation involves recognizing what is disturbing and using resources to counter a negative over-reaction. Calming techniques may already be used by the individual in mildly stressful situations or when they are self-absorbed and coping well. Worry beads, squeeze balls, tapping a foot, or using gross motor skills (heavy physical activity) might be comforting and decrease stress.

Younger individuals may have meltdowns in times of tiredness or incessant noise. AS adolescents commonly "self-medicate" in high stress situations and alcohol or drug taking can become strategies for coping. With maturity, they should recognize that some environments are likely to be exciting but provoke emotional overload. Developing independence brings responsibility to predict which environments are congruent with individual needs and to make healthy choices based on those needs.

Adolescents should understand how to modify the impact of AS traits on study or work. Study strategies might include headphones to exclude distracting noise. Working in an environment where there are less people and noise might be a priority. Calming environments and appropriate leisure activities (fishing, horse riding, solitary sports) can be explored for an individual with limited tolerance of high stimulus environments. Imagery and various types of meditative or relaxation exercises can be learned and practiced easily and effectively.

Adolescence is a time of transitions – between schools, from a protected environment to growing independence, from school peers to more mature friendships. There may be a move from home, a need to learn how to organize one's shopping and household demands, budgeting money, and so on. Change can be very threatening for the AS individual who enjoys familiarity. Anticipation of transitions provokes stress. Preparation can include predictions and rehearsal about what should be expected and practical ways of handling those things.

Because the AS individual is typically not self-reflective and finds his own and others' emotions confusing, self-regulation must include efforts to understand and deal appropriately with emotions. We have already established that the AS individual thinks "differently." Thoughts and emotions and behaviors are not independent. Thoughts cause feelings, feelings cause behavior. If we want to understand someone's behavior we need to look at their feelings. More than that, we need to acknowledge and accept the validity of their feelings, not tell them how they "should" be feeling. In supporting them, we can make them aware of their feelings, the connection between feelings and behavior, and our acceptance of their feelings.

When identifying emotions, context should be considered, along with likely triggers and associated physical cues. For example, a stomach ache or growing restlessness might be the best indicator that anxiety is being experienced. If it is understood that feelings of wanting to hit someone are an indicator of frustration or confusion, those feelings can be dealt with more appropriately. One of the most valuable contributions made by creative activity therapy is the opportunity to express feelings for which words cannot be found.

The parent and professional can introduce self-calming techniques. For example, before a session that involves creative activities, a routine of meditative or relaxation exercises can be used. Similarly, music or visual imagery can be used to deliberately introduce a different mood. The objective of such exercises is not just the immediate benefit of calming an individual for the session in hand, but illustrating effective techniques for changing mood and taking control of emotions rather than thoughtless reaction to external conditions.

ANXIETY, CONFIDENCE, ESTEEM, AND DEPRESSION

Anxiety, confidence, esteem, and depression are, not surprisingly, very much connected to each other. Stress from environment, expectations, sensory input, and so on cause anxiety to be high in most AS individuals. Many will appear not to be stressed at all. In fact, it is likely that they are shutting down in the face of everything that seems to rush at them – focusing on the bird outside the window rather than all the noise around them. Try to keep noise and chaos down to a reasonable level in a class or session or all efforts will be doomed to failure in the confusion.

As a consequence of difficulties with social interaction, eccentric ways of talking and dressing, and increasing sense of differences, the AS adolescent may suffer from low esteem and confidence. Telling your child that they are special and then packing them off to an unsympathetic school won't do the trick. Genuine self-esteem is not a product of words but of reality and experience. Try to give every opportunity to a teenager to develop and express his uniqueness in an environment that is sincerely appreciative of it. Older people are often more tolerant and appreciative of eccentricity than same age peers, and are more likely to be nurturing. AS individuals usually feel very comfortable with older people, perhaps for this reason.

Parents and professionals should be sensitive to a potential for depression, commonly experienced and manifested in different ways. Many teenagers are vulnerable to self-harm and bad choices when depressed, and for those who experience it early in life depression is likely to recur over the years. Depression sometimes results in suicide (the second or third most common cause of adolescent deaths worldwide). Another precursor to suicide is the use of alcohol or substance use, often a crude form of "self-medication." The importance of recognizing, understanding, and treating depression cannot be underestimated.

Depression is even more common for adolescents with Asperger's Syndrome, possibly because of the feelings of difference and isolation that they often experience. While there is no medication to decrease the experience of Asperger's Syndrome, medication may be required to reduce feelings of depression and the associated anxiety. Any suspicion of depression should also be clinically assessed for bipolar tendencies and manic, psychotic, or other features. Depressions differ in type and appropriate treatment. However, the possible impact and influence of any symptoms of depression should not be minimized. Symptoms and traits of depression include:

- general unhappiness, sadness and emptiness, loss of interest and pleasure, anxiety, crying (although some AS individuals tend to cry when overwhelmed with a rush of emotion if there is an inability to recognize and express emotions more "appropriately")

- constant irritability

- significant weight loss or gain

- frequent insomnia or hypersomnia

- agitated or notably slowed down behavior (if these are normal behavioral traits, look for changes)

- fatigue or loss of energy

- feelings of worthlessness or guilt

- diminished ability to think or concentrate

- indecisiveness

- recurrent thoughts of death or suicidal ideation

- self-hate and accusations, pessimism, hopelessness

- social withdrawal and a sense of failure.

Individuals with traits of Asperger's Syndrome often feel "different" from an early age but may not be able to identify why they are different. Feelings of anxiety, alienation, and desire to appear normal are likely to increase in adolescence as peers are less tolerant than they were in earlier years and often more worldly. Tony Attwood (1998) describes "wanting to be like others and have friends, and not knowing how to succeed" as the most common cause of depression.

The AS individual struggles to appear normal and perhaps develop relationships with people of the opposite gender. They may be falling back in their education. They may be forced to make compromises in expectations and choices in school and career goals. There may be a family history of depression (AS also has a tendency to occur more often in some families). Parental depression might be contributing to stress on the adolescent. Family dynamics cannot be discounted when assessing any child or adolescent.

Depression in AS individuals may be expressed through aggression and self-medication through alcohol. In their book on resilience and depression, authors Karen Reivich and Andrew Shatte (2002) point to depression being born from perception of a bleak future, a "pervasive sense of hopelessness" with associated negative thoughts and behaviors. In its early stages, depression can be effectively treated, but left untreated those thoughts and behaviors can have longlasting and negative repercussions (addictions, consequences of bad choices, and so on).

In summary, depression is a common and significant problem for adolescents. "Typical teenager" or "It is just a stage he's going through" are not helpful responses. Parents and adolescents would benefit from joining a local support group, connecting to others with similar experiences, asking for recommendations to good local professionals, and learning about resources available to them.

PSYCHOTHERAPEUTIC TREATMENT OF DEPRESSION

Depression can originate from physiology or chemical imbalances, environmental stress, and/or an individual's thoughts and behaviors. For a long time it has been the belief that the most effective treatment for clinical depression is a combination of medication and psychotherapy. However, a comprehensive book summarizing results of multiple meta-analyses of successful treatments for depression (Beutler, Clarkin and Bongar 2000) suggests that psychotherapy seems to be significantly more effective than pharmacotherapy. In fact, psychotherapy alone may be superior to a combined approach. Certainly, the effects of psychotherapy are more effective over a long time than medication because of the preventative (vs. "cure") approach.

Cognitive behavior modification is particularly effective in addressing depression. It addresses specific issues that are important for the individual and can increase coping and adaptive skills, particularly in learning how to manage relevant issues, and reduce overwhelming experiences of emotion such as sadness, anxiety, and frustration. Therapy also offers opportunities to learn and practice skills to manage depressive reactions to future events and potential situations.

In meta-analyses of different types of therapies it has been found that individual and group therapies are equally effective – in fact, group therapy may be slightly more effective. This is good news for the AS individual because group therapy can simultaneously address other issues relevant to Asperger's Syndrome (practice of social skills, goal setting, problem solving). Group therapy is generally less expensive than individual therapy – an important consideration because AS support is typically based on long-term practice of behavior and skills more than short-term solutions. That said, some personal issues may arise that are better handled in individual and family therapy.

Given that group therapy is as effective as individual therapy, working with art in groups offers infinite opportunities for support. When treating depression in Asperger adolescents, we fall back on the principles that have been shown to build resilience. Self-awareness provides the basic foundation from which changes can be made. The resilience model also holds that an active engagement and involvement with something other than one's self (such as contributing to a group, group goals and activities) will act to reduce depression.

Art and creative therapies can be designed to explore individuality and develop self-awareness – strengths, weaknesses, perceptions, reactions, thoughts and beliefs about people and situations, and a supportive context in which to challenge any unrealistic thoughts and beliefs. It is through these exercises that goals, motivations, tasks, and meaning emerge – all of which can play a part in countering depression. Art provides a language of communication, not just in clarifying self-awareness but communicating information to other people. As an example, I asked a young boy to draw the shape of Asperger's Syndrome for me. He drew a one line scribble and told me it was "a man-eating plant – that's what Asperger's is."

"It might be a boy-eating plant," I responded.

"No," he said. "Boys are very active and thin and can slip out sideways." (This child was extremely animated and easily agitated.) "But then," he added sadly, adding strokes to the original drawing, "the plant has feelers that pull the boy back in."

The picture gave the language to describe the feelings and, perhaps, behavior. Cognitive behavioral therapy (CBT) is generally the most effective way to change thoughts and behavior. Another approach is to change the behavior which will produce a change in outcome – and thoughts about the behavior will change as a consequence. For example, if an adolescent has difficulty in changing thoughts of resentment and anger toward a classmate, initiating a different behavior such as including the person in question in an invitation to a game or the movies may produce a friendlier experience with the person, and changed thoughts about them.

A group is useful for changing patterns of thinking (cognitive behavioral therapy) because when experiences and issues are shared, often other group members can contribute to a discussion of alternative ways of thinking and being, check the reality of thoughts, and support efforts to change behavior. Again, self-awareness plays an important role in effective CBT treatment. Creative therapies help stimulate new ways of thinking about ourselves and our roles rather than reiterating the "old stories."

In conclusion, self-awareness is a work in progress, in concert with life itself. Creative expression – through writing, painting, visual and auditory forms of representation – cannot be overestimated in its value as an enjoyable but insightful resource for the individual to become aware of and be responsible for their emotions, thoughts, and behaviors.

## Social difficulties and connecting with the world

The way we think impacts on our behavior and subsequent outcomes. Ultimately, the thought-processing difficulties for AS adolescents will affect social interaction – with friends and family; at school, college, work; and when living with other people. Appropriate social interaction and negotiation may be stressful for the individual moving from the familiarity and comfort of home to independence in the outside world. Let's briefly look at the unique difficulties an AS individual may have in social interactions.

### Theory of mind

Related to symbolic thought is theory of mind, understanding the mental states and attitudes of other people. Just as symbolic thinking allows the individual to think about something without actually experiencing it, theory of mind allows the individual to understand other people's perspectives, beliefs, desires, and possible intentions. Lacking theory of mind has far-reaching consequences for social skills and ability to interact with the world. Individuals with AS see the world from their own perspective. They often fail to recognize that other people have different perspectives, feelings, thoughts, and ways of behaving. Honesty, open-handedness, and lack of deceit are among the attractive traits typically seen in Asperger's Syndrome. But it can also mean that these individuals are naïve and taken advantage of. They may not be able to predict the behavior of others or understand their motives. This can have implications for the handling of sexual and/or threatening situations that may arise for adolescents.

With the assumption that other people share the same feelings there is often no attempt by people with AS to explain their own thoughts, behavior, or intentions. They may not be able to make connections between their behavior and other people's reaction to that behavior. When one adolescent was asked why he was unjustifiably violent, he replied, "I wondered what it would feel like. It didn't feel good so I won't do it again." The response was honest, logical, and naïve, without malice, yet reflecting a lack of awareness of the perspective of the person on the receiving end of the violence.

The AS individual may give the impression of having little empathy for others but that isn't accurate. If they are aware of the distress of another person, they will probably be sincerely concerned. Becoming aware and attuned to someone else's feelings and expressing concern appropriately are difficult. Facial cues are often not understood, and in language subtleties or implied meaning will be missed. Unless cues have been learned, sarcasm, joking, and teasing can be misunderstood. There is often a lack of ability to read between the lines or body language, or pick up on cues such as tone of voice. An example of this is one child who asked his mother why she was yelling at him. "Because I'm angry at you." His reply of "Well, why didn't you tell me?" is a typical example of literal interpretation and simple logic.

In his account of life as a young adolescent with Asperger's Syndrome, Luke Jackson (2002) writes that "precise parents make cheerful children." Instructions to children should be given clearly and in a way that can't be misconstrued if interpreted literally. Don't assume that individuals are aware of the reasons for activities at home and school, or the expectations and demands made of them. Making connections or seeing the relevance between one situation and another cannot be assumed. A parent or teacher might seem to be always angry at an AS individual. Frustration should be explained in simple terms. Connections should be made between the immediate context and underlying reasons. For example, "I am angry because you are late" will not be as effective as "When you are late, I worry that you may be hurt. It is important for your safety that I know where you are after you leave school. If you ever change your plans and will be late, you must call me."

Support can be given to developing theory of mind through discussion and developing understanding of visual language by role playing, and exploring other people's possible perspectives. Imaginary play and practice of social communication also allow initiation of novel situations.

### Social interaction

A support group offers opportunities for practicing social skills. A group allows members to enjoy meeting others with similar interests and concerns, and may lead to developing genuine friendships around subjects of shared interest. Integrating social situations such as outings to a coffee shop, bookshop, or restaurant can also be helpful. Appropriate behavior in nurturing friendships has a better chance of being generalized from active participation in the group to school, work, and the "outside world" than theory alone.

Building a sense of friendship and teamwork entails encouraging team members to acknowledge the value of other members, listen to their experiences and interests, and not dominate the floor. The quiet individual should be encouraged to contribute and their contribution validated. Developing social skills includes asking questions of another group member, exhibiting interest in them and their lives, discussion of appropriate social manners (should a young man open a door for a young lady?), appropriate body space and eye contact, topics of conversation appropriate to the type of acquaintance, and role playing or practicing social situations that might arise (asking someone on a date, a job interview).

Social outings provide opportunities for discussion of expectations, construction of desired outcomes, practicing appropriate and reciprocal conversation. Feedback after these experiences is important, from different perspectives. (What happened to you? How do you think the waitress felt when you…? Sean didn't say much all night – how do you think he was feeling? What could you have said to make him feel more included in the group?)

Sometimes videotaping social interaction effectively reinforces what is intellectually known. Replaying videotape allows different perspectives to be taken. (Did you see how David was talking about his model cars and you interrupted? Do you notice that you spoke for 90 percent of the time and it looks like a one-man conversation?) Another technique is to turn the sound down on the television and discuss what scenario may be taking place through interpretation of body language. (Look how he's turning his body away – does he look interested in the conversation?)

It is important to help the individual make the connection to different contexts. What is appropriate behavior and language in one context is not appropriate in another. This learning can be visually supported with self-made cue cards, social stories, and cartoons. Use art or drama to support learning social skills. It allows time for the individual to process the information without being overwhelmed by verbal instructions, and may be more easily retrieved from memory in different real-life contexts because of the visual cues.

What else does a support group with art and creative activities offer? Individuals with AS often have difficulties with taking turns, being polite, and respecting social conventions and manners. Participating in an interactive art group offers opportunities for team building, sharing, cooperating, and turn taking.

Given the difficulties with cognitive processing for AS individuals, and subsequent difficulties in interacting with other people, what are useful techniques that can be used to help facilitate communications skills and resilience? A most effective therapeutic strategy is cognitive behavioral – changing thoughts to change behavior. The core of cognitive behavioral therapy is as simple as ABC. An individual can be taught to apply ABC technique in daily problem solving and reaction to stressful situations:

**A**  *Adversity* or *Antecedent* (problem, difficult situation or relationship)

**B**  *Beliefs* and thoughts about the adversity/situation/relationship that is causing stress

**C**  *Consequences* (thoughts and behaviors).

Shelley is leaving school soon and is anxious about the transition to college. She has never liked change and she is so unhappy about this that it is starting to affect her grades. In a group, or with a parent or therapist, Shelley's beliefs about the transition can be explored. She knows she is clumsy with other people, often says the wrong thing, and sometimes doesn't connect faces to previous conversations or recognize people a second time.

The consequences of these thoughts are that Shelley believes people will consider her to be stupid; she will be excluded, alone, and miserable.

Stop all thoughts! Just because she thinks these things doesn't mean they are true. But unless some changes are made to Shelley's thoughts about going to college, there is a possibility that she will keep to herself, remain isolated, and her fears will be a self-fulfilling prophecy.

Consequences are paired with beliefs and a change in one will effect a change in the other. With help, the validity and absolute nature of her beliefs can be questioned. Shelley can explore the reality of going to college from different perspectives: What does she imagine the college experience to be like? Why does she think it will be so? Where will she be spending most of her time? How would she like it to be? What are five things she would like to get out of college? What are her long-term goals and how can the college experience fit into that? If making friends is so important, what is she looking for in friendship? Where is she likely to find such people?

Consequently, Shelley may change her belief from thinking a positive college experience will be founded on being liked by others to focusing on opportunities to work on the college newspaper. She loves research and eventually would like to work in an area where she can help others. The consequences of the change in belief ("college is an opportunity to extend my knowledge about research and writing") means that she is now productive, working with her strengths, and keeping company with like-minded people. She is much happier than first imagined.

In their book *The Resilience Factor*, Reivich and Shatte (2002) have identified eight common thinking traps to be watchful for. Many are highly pertinent to Asperger's Syndrome and include:

- jumping to conclusions (highly likely with AS because of reliance on past experience and lack of awareness of alternative perspectives)

- tunnel vision (particularly appropriate for AS individuals who can focus on details at the expense of the "bigger picture")

- magnifying and minimizing (catastrophic or all-or-nothing thinking – everything turns bad for me, this always happens to me, it is never going to get better – all hallmarks of depression)

- personalizing (also highly appropriate for AS adolescents who tend to see themselves as the center of the universe and everything relating to him or herself – attributing problems to oneself instead of seeing the "bigger picture")

- externalizing (blaming others for a situation because of the inability to see how one can effect some change and control)

- overgeneralizing (another particularly pertinent trap for AS adolescents – just because a particular behavior was successful in achieving an outcome in the past doesn't mean it will be successful with other people or in another context)

- mind reading or believing we know what other people are thinking. For the non-AS individual, this may have a slightly different meaning than for AS individuals who tend to assume that others think like themselves, have the same motivations and reasoning

- emotional reasoning – "drawing false conclusions about the nature of the world based on emotional state" (remembering Shelley, the anxiety of social interaction at college contributed to her belief that it would be a negative experience; and as a result she might reduce her anxiety by staying in her room and becoming more isolated. AS adolescents benefit from understanding their emotions and likely emotional reactions).

Underlying beliefs might be the product of upbringing or, especially in the case of AS individuals, born from just one relatively unimportant but significant experience which has skewed an attitude or belief.

One adolescent was resentful of having to see a therapist although he was clearly having problems at school and was being assessed for Asperger's Syndrome. After some investigation it emerged that he associated the words "Asperger's Syndrome" with Acquired Immune Deficiency Syndrome, or AIDS. Identifying the confusion allowed clarification of what a syndrome is (a collection of traits). Thoughts and beliefs about a diagnosis of Asperger's Syndrome were changed from negative to positive (a diagnosis enabled an understanding of the nature and impact of Asperger's Syndrome, and information is power). The change in thoughts effected a change in behavior and the young man became a cooperative partner in a support group.

It is not in the nature of most people to argue with themselves or to question the validity of what they think or believe. In fact, it seems to be a normal tendency to look for evidence to support beliefs which we've already acquired. A valuable skill is to take any problematic situation as a cue to explore alternative ways of thinking. Ask members of a group to contribute to a list of problematic situations. Then as a group, question the thoughts and beliefs that support the belief that the situation is a "problem." Refer to Reivich and Shatte's list of eight "thinking traps" (2002) to break down negative beliefs. Encourage group members to get into the habit of checking other perspectives before coming to a conclusion.

Losing your calm, losing your head, and losing your focus have been identified by Reivich and Shatte (2002) as "draining reserves of resilience." These are typical behaviors of adolescents with AS traits. As well as antecedent thoughts, intrusive thoughts can be a problem. AS individuals sometimes experience pictures flashing through their heads, often go off on tangents, and are easily distracted. Logic can also be rudely interrupted by emotional reactions with typically negative or defensive thoughts (sometimes manifested in aggressive behavior to regain control or put people at a distance).

Most individuals benefit from learning self-calming strategies – visualization, yoga, controlled breathing, progressive relaxation, exercise, and refocusing techniques are just a few. Support groups are most effective when they include physically calming exercises, both as an introduction to a session in order for optimum benefit, or as a conclusion to learn skills to utilize in stress-provoking situations during the week. Groups can regularly provide opportunities for members to give examples of their self-regulation during the week, for which they should be commended.

## Connectedness

Connectedness is a cornerstone to a happy and healthy life. This chapter looks at how it can be expected to impact on the life of an adolescent with AS. Asperger's Syndrome is a collection of traits that can and will be modified throughout life. Sometimes a child who has been diagnosed as having very strong traits can modify them so much over time, experience, and exposure that DSM diagnosis criteria may not be met when they are older. On the other hand, with the independence of adulthood, traits may become more exaggerated and the individual increasingly perceived as eccentric. Other than self-awareness, the single most influential factor in lifelong modification may be "connectedness."

When living in a situation where connectedness with other people forces behavior modification and compromise – through living with others, working with others, traveling, and so on – the individual usually adapts and exhibits less Asperger traits (although underlying ways of thinking are difficult to modify such as literal thinking, difficulty in organization). Those individuals who, for one reason or another, find themselves in a position of relative isolation – living at home, not working, or working in a protected environment that requires limited contact with other people – are not required to modify their behavior. There will be less effort, for example, to dress like other people or socialize or broaden interests.

It is important that adolescents themselves understand the importance of connectedness. It broadens the potential to live full and satisfying lives. There may be a tendency to avoid other people because of the effort and discomfort involved but the effort is worthwhile. Being the star of their own show, a common Asperger trait is to underestimate the positive and negative impact that other people and experiences can have. It is inevitable that the connections – or lack of them – mold us and our lives. Encourage awareness and responsibility for connections made.

Adolescent development is a product of experience. As the child matures, experiences and feedback from others will help define self-concept, beliefs, and choices. Naturally, when connections play such an important role in the way we develop, it is beneficial to take some control in choosing who we spend our time with. Unfortunately, some AS adolescents will make poor choices because of lack of discrimination and an inability to read the correct motivations of other people.

What sort of connections are most helpful for AS individuals? It can be easier to relate to older people than peers, and younger, concrete-thinking children are less complicated, more accepting. There are benefits in spending time with older relatives or professionals who share similar interests. Often, older family members will have the patience and concern to help AS adolescents explore different activities, and in so doing build caring, reciprocal relationships. AS individuals are typically attached to their families and the familiarity of home. It is the ideal space for realistic but resilient development.

The resilience model suggests that identifying our strengths is a useful factor. Taking interests – even obsessions – and finding groups of similarly minded people will be useful. Not only is the individual making pleasant social contacts, but also the interaction is likely to be more heartfelt because of the shared interests. Self-esteem may develop out of mutual respect in such a group and the interest might even be developed to the extent that it plays a part in career choice. The AS individual is not only connecting to other people in this context but also given the opportunity to connect with a unique and valued part of self.

For all individuals, connectedness is beneficial when the individual perceives himself or herself to be part of a greater whole (nationality, culture, school, interest group, and so on). It is beneficial when it provides opportunities to lose a sense of separateness and enter a state of "flow" (work, conversation with other people, challenging interests); a genuine and emotional connectedness with others (through a support group, with caring family members, or in a small group of friends); when connectedness has a two-way street character (the individual is contributing back to the connection; giving, not just taking from it; listening, not just speaking; teaching, not just learning).

Connectedness plays an important role in development of "meaning" and purpose in life. Personal values provide direction and a foundation for resilience. Those with AS usually have a natural sense of fairness and concern for justice. If they could afford to live apart from other people, their sense of natural justice and truth might never be questioned. Unfortunately, real life isn't always clear cut and the concrete way of thinking, typical of Asperger's Syndrome, will not be enough when an experience or concept cannot be explained in logical concrete terms. Understanding life from a purely egocentric perspective will result in a rigid, non-adaptive way of thinking.

Temple Grandin has written about the Asperger perspective of concepts such as "beauty, justice and truth." It is difficult for her to understand a concept unless it is paired with a picture or real-life example. She can associate the concept of beauty through a picture of a sunset, and associates justice with courtroom movies and scenes on television. The concrete explanation for quantum theory contributes more to her belief in God and a "cosmic consciousness" than any esoteric argument. For the Asperger individual, the acquisition of "meaning," and the resilience that it affords, is likely to be a product of concrete fact, real or observed experience.

Yet the experiential and concrete perspective of the Asperger individual does fail to support many experiences. Being able to make connections to other people or something beyond themselves is one of the strongest sources of support and resilience. Connecting to other people – hearing their experiences, building genuine empathy – is important. Many children with strong traits of Asperger's Syndrome modify those traits and their values considerably as they mature, through connections with other people, observing and learning from other people's experiences.

Connecting to the world through interests and work is important. "Being engaged in life's tasks" (Frankl 1997) and engaging in life to the extent that self-consciousness is lost (Csikszentmihalyi 1997) offer practical and pragmatic paths of connectedness and resilience to the AS individual. In addition, development of the AS adolescent will benefit from connecting in different spheres that add to the complexity of the self-concept. Even if it is difficult for him or her to be employed, valuable experiences can be gained from voluntary work, taking part in community activities, and so on. Just as practice of social skills makes them easier to apply, so connective experiences to others introduce adaptive ways of thinking and being.

Places to make meaningful connections might occur at school with peers and teachers; within the family (immediate and extended); in the community with neighbors or membership of groups such as churches, recreational or sporting groups; cultural activities that may be available. Professionals can help identify situations where the AS individual has something valuable to offer and his or her contribution will be acknowledged.

## How does the SEL model support AS adolescents in their interaction with others?

Social and Emotional Learning (SEL) promotes principles toward making positive and responsible choices. The AS adolescent is moving away from his family, ideally toward independent living and possibly marriage. This is a time for setting goals, discussing the process of reaching goals, taking responsibility for choices, along with an awareness of the repercussions of different choices. Group support is an excellent resource in this area. Parents may inadvertently minimize or not be aware of some of the challenges that AS peers would relate to.

The fact that thoughts are not necessarily valid or true is especially pertinent for the AS adolescent. Establishing a support network of people with whom the "truth" can be tested would benefit the adolescent. Having a non-AS buddy to help negotiate through school, college, and social situations would be extremely helpful. Being able to check alternative perspectives with non-AS people will open self-imposed boundaries for the AS adolescent. Encouragement to go beyond the comforts of familiarity to try new things, such as traveling, can also bring many rewards.

Nothing teaches as well as exposure and experience. The SEL focus on values should come easily to the AS adolescent who typically has an innate desire for justice and integrity. However, the mistaken assumption that others will also act fairly may bring disappointment. Learning cues to identify insincerity and false friendship is helpful.

The principle of subjective perspectives – the personal bias that everybody has due to their own experience – is particularly relevant to the cognitive processing weaknesses of the AS adolescent. Ongoing self-consciousness is necessary to identify motivations, underlying beliefs, and "meaningfulness" of behavior, another principle of the SEL model. Positive development requires an ability to adapt and modify behavior without compromising integrity. Ability to express oneself appropriately is also important in this area. Practice through role play of specific situations such as a student or worker negotiating and compromising in a conversation.

Sexuality may become an area of concern sooner or later and the AS adolescent would benefit from having a safe, supportive environment in which to discuss those issues openly. Social and emotional skills include skills in meeting other people, appropriate topics and course of conversation, possible motivations, agendas, and expectations of other people, how to pick up on cues in what other people might be thinking, awareness of responsibilities in a relationship, dealing with the moral issues of sexuality, emotions, how perspectives and values might differ between people, how to react to different situations, and practicing ways of asserting oneself. Awareness of sexual and dating safety is very important and should be addressed and discussed openly.

Finally, SEL refers not only to interacting with other people with respect but also managing oneself and working toward goals with negotiation skills. One of the central goals in supporting the AS individual is to teach skills which allow an independence toward a unique and fulfilling life. Self-awareness, emotional, and communicative skills are not just goals in themselves but provide a foundation in reaching that goal of self-actualization.

## Creative learning

Jonathan Cohen (2001) identified creative learning as being extremely useful in building social and emotional skills. It is particularly useful for building skills in those with Asperger's Syndrome. Creativity is a cornerstone of integrative and adaptive thinking, for making social and emotional connections, using language and representational thought, facilitating novel and unconventional expression, exploring ideas, and developing concepts.

The creative process employs goal setting and holistic, integrative thinking – seeing the big picture and working towards it. Through creativity, new perspectives are realized, ideas generated, goals set, and all varieties of solutions found. Creativity breaks through rigidity and the safety of familiar boundaries. It is a new way of seeing and a door to freedom, resilience, and a positive life for adolescents with Asperger's Syndrome.

# Part II

# Creative Activities

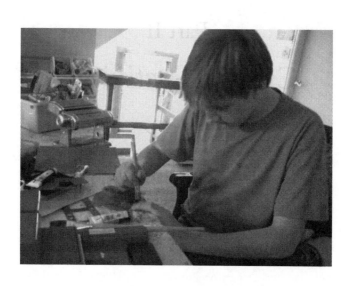

# CHAPTER 4

# Groups

## A word about groups

The most effective support for AS usually comes from long-term interaction and learning in groups. The "little professor" demeanor of many AS individuals means that they relate very well in a one-to-one relationship with an adult counselor. It is in a group context with their peers that more problems are likely to become salient and more learning is likely to occur. It is also more financially feasible than ongoing individual support.

As the AS individual develops there will be changing needs and groups can be found or formed to meet needs accordingly. Social skills building with concrete behavioral strategies form the basis of most AS support groups for younger ages. Because of the nature of learning and practicing social skills, each person needs individual attention and cueing. No more than six participants is advisable, with a comfortable number of co-facilitators (approximate ratio of 1:2). A token economy may be set up to reinforce behavior. An hour is an appropriate length of time for younger groups.

At high school, different issues will emerge. Ideally, groups run longer than an hour to meet individual needs and the different character of older groups. Creative activities suggested in this book will be more effective if groups run longer than an hour, using them to introduce shared experiences and build relationships.

Individuals may discuss their personal experiences and expectations on issues such as relationships, exploring career possibilities, fears of entering college or the workforce, developing independence. Groups offer opportunities to meet others with similar experiences and lessen feelings of isolation or social discomfort. These groups can be slightly larger than the younger groups but small enough for all members to freely contribute to a discussion.

A central goal of older groups could be to encourage cohesiveness that may extend beyond the context of a support group to form friendships and a social network.

An open format is necessary for an ongoing group. This has advantages because new members can be introduced at any time and some members will drop out as they grow too old for the group, take a vacation, and so on. Disadvantages include difficulties in maintaining cohesiveness when there is a fluctuating membership and a new member may initially feel like an outsider. Facilitators can counter this through using variations on introduction techniques when new members are introduced.

Because social graces are not a strong point for AS, "rules" and behavioral expectations should be clear. It is important to periodically remind or discuss the issue of confidentiality with group members. A common behavior is the tendency to go off at tangents or for the conversation to be dominated by one person, loudness, or a lack of order. The group may jointly decide on a hand signal or cue (such as a T formed with the hands) indicating "time out" to curtail these disruptions. Being rule lovers, group members may be quicker than the facilitator to get a discussion off a tangent and back on track. Engaging group members to form their own group rules will ensure greater enthusiasm in keeping them.

Participation should be encouraged through open questioning, doing "rounds" for comments on a topic, invitations to share experiences, or breaking the group into dyads (two members) for particular exercises to encourage active participation. If a group member is quiet and not keen to contribute, that should be respected. At all times, in every group, participants must be aware that they have the choice to participate or not in an activity. Respond with a comment such as "That's okay. We all feel like standing back sometimes. Maybe you'll share in the activity next week."

Some individuals will feel safer just observing and that can be an effective learning strategy. The importance of an environment that is comfortable and safe and where everybody's individuality is respected cannot be underestimated.

## Setting up for art-related creative activities

There are many excellent art/craft books that give step-by-step instructions for making specific objects. However, the activities in this book encourage original and individual expression, spontaneity, and self-organization. The least intimidating way to facilitate spontaneity and originality is as follows:

- excessive variety, types, and colors of available materials – what is inspiring to one person will not be inspiring to another
- fewer instructions and more visual, concrete examples of potential ways to use materials
- assurance that there is no one "right" way to do anything and that the goal is to be yourself not someone else, no matter how clever they are.

Many art-related activities in this book require materials and techniques for expressive art. Expressive art relies on access to a broad collection of materials including paint, papers, metal, fabric, photos, and so on. Throw a mixture of things into the middle of the table (the more versatile expressive and symbolic potential the better). Unique combinations will emerge that you would never have thought of. There are suggestions for collage materials and medium in Chapter 8.

## Sampler of colors and effects

Provide a "sampler" of paints and different effects, showing different techniques, for easy visual referral without taking a lot of instruction time. Accompany the sampler with a visual cue (photocopy) of the sequence of relevant steps. Pictures and examples are worth a thousand words.

## Color chart

Leave a color chart/sampler in the middle of the table, and casually refer to it – three basic colors, with mixes leaning toward one of the other two. Lack of understanding of color causes some trepidation for a lot of people yet it can be demystified very easily. Having a wide variety of ready-made colors available will also make things simpler.

## Words

Words can be introduced through hand printing or writing, stamps, computer fonts and graphics, or hand-held dynamo (office supplies). If words are relevant but participants don't want to put words into their art exercises, they can be written on a separate piece of paper. It is in the process of creativity that new ways of seeing and thinking about things are realized – ideas, associations, and related words. Words that have been written down during the process can be explored further later.

*Beginning*

It can be very difficult to start something, especially when the finished product is not defined and concrete steps cannot be followed. These activities provide general instructions and structure (theme, examples of possibilities, basic instructions), yet broad potential for individualization (available materials, many ways to be used and interpreted) and support while the process unfolds.

Yes, all the potential can be overwhelming. Some individuals will need more help than others to get started. Technical mistakes will be made. Part of the process is embracing the potential of many possibilities, choosing a road, putting one step in front of the other, problem solving, appreciating and being appreciated for the courage and choices, the wonder of inventiveness, imagination, creativity – the way things "work out."

*Techniques and media*

When choosing appropriate techniques and media, assessment of personal likes and dislikes and engaging the cooperation of the individual in setting goals is essential. When designing specific activities, consider and integrate the following factors:

- developmental stage of the individuals (motor skills, cognitive)
- interests of the individuals (relevant to gender, sensory preferences, personality, relationship style, obsessions)
- available and appropriate medium, time, space, resources.

When activities are presented, different forms of media are suggested. For example, one activity in Frustration and anger management (6.34) uses "expressive art, drama, puppetry." Expressive art relates to paint, collage, any type of media which allows direct and spontaneous self-expression. Another activity under the same theme (6.33) uses "visualization." This theme can be explored endlessly through unique combinations of different media, frameworks, developmental stages, and so on. An ongoing process over a number of sessions may combine and relate one theme to other themes. Activities may be focused on one individual or provide material for group discussion and comparison. They can be modified for maturing and mature ages.

Being conscious of creative variations and possibilities allows the facilitator to be true to underlying goals and principles yet flexible and able to change direction within a session if appropriate. It is not necessary to be sophisticated in knowledge of art techniques but be familiar enough to understand what is involved with using different mediums, to have the correct tools and materials, and be able to impart technical information to students in a familiar, relatively simple way without letting it become the focus point of the group. From the outset, it should be made clear that this is not an art class. The paint/clay/whatever is to be used as an enjoyable alternative way to complete the exploratory task of the day.

An introduction to the nuts and bolts of art techniques is in Chapter 8. For our purposes – keeping it simple and honest – this should provide the basics. Unfortunately, we live in a world where one has to be brave to be naïve. There seems to be an implicit rule that if we're not good at something we have no business doing it and many people are highly self-critical of their own work. I have often made the point with group members that Anne Frank was not a writer – what she had to say was more important than the way she said it. Appreciation for self-disclosure should be expressed. The need for confidentiality within the group should be restated on a regular basis.

Focus on feelings when discussing a theme, and encourage new ways of saying or seeing something that may habitually have used an old "script." Lines, shapes, colors, textures all contribute to self-expression and can be more informative than the image itself. Don't make assumptions about the meaning of any mark and resist making your own interpretations of someone's work. Take an approach similar to "That's a heavy line…it all looks very dark…an interesting corner. What do you think that means? What does that mean to you?" Avoid making value judgments.

In conclusion, activities are presented in categories of developmental themes and principles. They are meant as starting points and examples. The most effective interventions will be individualized by the parent or mentor through integration of themes/questions with real-life applicability. Designing and modifying expressive therapies through these endless combinations will offer more flexibility and relevance than following a set of non-personalized exercises.

## Themes and activities

We are the sum of all our experiences. (Unknown)

Individuals with AS traits often appear to be extremely high-functioning. A teenager may have been diagnosed earlier in life and great strides have been made, he or she has been mainstreamed in education and is now realistically anticipating working and living independently. Indeed, it may be just a few traits that can now be easily identified. To new friends and acquaintances, this individual may seem quirky, eccentric, intelligent. Little indicates that the teenager with Asperger's still feels different, even alienated, and struggles daily with things taken for granted by other people.

These activities are generally aimed for the adolescent and young person who appears to be functioning very well while still struggling with some fundamental issues. Those issues may manifest in a lack of organization, social clumsiness, or poor choices. There may be alienation, a lack of confidence, depression, and avoidance situations where potential can be developed.

Activities should be tailored to individual needs and skill levels. Activities also have to cater to individual differences in circumstances and likes and dislikes. A particular character will emerge from each group – some will prefer drama, some will be quieter and less demonstrative. Activities will be more engaging and effective when they are designed to meet personal preferences.

### Framework

The framework for designing effective support rests on the three broad areas where traits of Asperger's Syndrome can be expected to cause difficulties.

1. Conceptual and cognitive processing; semantic and pragmatic weaknesses; imagination.

2. Self-awareness and self-related skills: emotion, depression, anxiety, emotional self-regulation.

3. Social difficulties and connecting with the world.

### Objectives

The objectives of the activities are drawn from the principles of Positive Psychology and Social Emotional Learning (SEL). For example, typical AS traits include difficulties in organization (Chapter 6) and appropriate social interaction (Chapter 7). Both Positive Psychology and SEL emphasize the importance of making meaningful connections with other people for positive development. Needs and goals can be integrated in objectives of activities such as Plan a party (5.5) and Building relationships #4 (7.34).

In these particular activities, the individual takes practical steps to organize a party, learns and rehearses appropriate social skills at a party, and may form good relationships with people in the group when this activity is practiced. In this way, activities are introduced to support the whole individual, within a framework that promotes positive development, rather than simply focusing on modifying problematic traits.

## Implementation of the objectives and activities

The implementation of the objectives and activities will depend on individual differences, access to resources, and appropriateness of therapy. The group facilitator is encouraged to pull different techniques from different areas of the book, to modify them and generate new ideas for application.

The activities are presented in a way that can be adapted to different ages. Techniques and activities can be modified according to skill level and materials and time available. For example, a group that is cohesive may be enthusiastic about doing a community activity together. Another group may prefer activities where everyone does their own thing within the group.

Within the group there will be individual differences. In activities requiring "expressive art" (painting, collage, etc.) one member may habitually finish quickly while others take more time. In this case, suggest making something with the art. The "wrapping technique" in Chapter 8 describes how a piece of paper or fabric can be wrapped around a board or three-dimensional object quite simply, extending the same project as needed. A piece of paper suddenly becomes a book cover or a puppet.

Some AS individuals will prefer "making something" rather than doing an activity purely for its expressive value. Variations on making something are endless. They keep the individual engaged in an ongoing process and do not compromise the integrity of the objective. In fact, sometimes it is the creativity that comes with problem solving in finishing a piece that provides new and different information to work with. A list of things to "make" is also included in Chapter 8.

## Self-expression

Completing the project or activity is not as important as the opportunity it gives to be self-expressive. Self-expression is not fully realized until the individual becomes conscious of their feelings toward a theme or issues that emerge. Discussion during and at the end of a session is more important than anything made. This is the time when self-realization becomes focused and purposeful, is validated, and may be extended further into discussion of associations, new learning, reinforcement of something already learned, goals.

The suggestions for discussion and questions can of course be para-phrased and adapted to the language interests and skill levels of different groups.

Despite group differences, it is suggested that special activities or "rituals" are used for Introductions (4.1, 4.2) and Saying goodbye (4.3). A common trait of AS is the appreciation of activities that are clearly defined with a beginning and an end. Another trait is the fondness for familiarity. It benefits nearly all groups and all ages to regularly begin sessions with a relaxation exercise (see 6.37 and 6.38).

### Themes

A set of activities related to one theme can be self-reinforcing over four to six weeks, before moving to another theme. Common to all themes, activities relate to social interaction, communication, and imagination. The following should be integrated informally and reinforced in different forms in every session:

- relaxation (self-awareness, stress relief, and self-regulation)
- relationships (in groups – teamwork, cooperation and compromise, reciprocity and friendship building, appropriate conversation, turn taking, space, social rules, etc.)
- novel ways of seeing, improving, and reinforcing learning in different contexts (generalizing, adapting)
- enjoying things that can normally be demanding and disliked (e.g. fine motor skill and coordination activity – enjoy rather than be outcome oriented)
- non-academic learning and new, unfamiliar things (activities, media), encouraging curiosity and creative expression (flexibility, adaptability)
- awareness and enhancement of personal strengths; commendation for strengths.

## Beyond Asperger's Syndrome

As mentioned earlier, individuals with AS will experience most of the transitions and difficulties experienced by those without AS. Themes will be presented that relate to issues relevant to all adolescents and young adults, not just those with Asperger's Syndrome.

In addition, some strengths and traits contribute to a happy and resilient development for those with and without Asperger's (curiosity, social and emotional intelligence, self-control, gratitude, playfulness, etc.). Some activity themes will focus on development of these positive traits rather than purely AS traits.

Examples of general but important themes are "my family", "good memories", "future directions", "facets of self", "connectedness to friends" and "a secret place". There may be a continuity in themes – the "past" theme of last week may be related to expectations for the "future" theme of this week; or connections made between perceptions of self from previous weeks and current exploration of relationships with others.

It is important that participants are made aware of the objective of each activity, how the objective relates to them and how the principles within the activity can be generalized to real life. Introduce the underlying concept and justification for the exercise. Education, responsibility and empowerment in making choices should underlie the goals of support for adolescents and young adults.

Staying on one theme, in different forms, is valuable. Self-awareness is the single most important theme. Offering opportunities for it to be explored differently through different media is likely to produce more unique, comprehensive and insightful experiences than just one exercise. Some themes, such as loss and grief, take time to process. Sometimes it emerges that an apparently simple subject has conflicting or contradictory emotions, and they take time to be realized, expressed, acknowledged and integrated.

Most of the following exercises were derived specifically for this book, integrating the principles above. Some are drawn from books which are credited. A few have been used in different contexts over a number of years but I do not know of their origin. My apologies for not always being able to give credit where it is due, when the source of exercises has been lost along the way.

## 4.1 Introductions #1
Picture interpretation.

### Objective
Introduce self to others.

### Implementation

1.  Take pictures from magazines that include people, things, situations, places, different medium, different perspectives, different moods. Some should be abstract or surreal – leave room for personal interpretation.

2.  Lay the pictures haphazardly on a table. Depending on the maturity level of the group, model by introducing yourself through a picture. "This picture of a … reminds me of myself. It is used as … and I feel that people treat me like that sometimes. … is hidden and there are hidden parts of myself. The colors appeal to me because they look like … And I think that's a part of my personality."

3.  Suggest that group members pick a picture that they feel represents them in some way. Invite them to introduce themselves through the picture they have chosen. If there is hesitancy, suggest a round. If a member is reluctant even after encouragement, respect their right to withdraw at any time.

### NOTE

This exercise can be used to introduce symbolism, is effective in introducing fragments of information that may not otherwise be brought up in a conventional introduction. It goes beyond name and school details and allows introductions to be elaborated in a direction that the participant perceives themselves or would like others to perceive them. It invites the participant to share as much as they wish with others without requiring eye contact (they can look at the picture while making the introduction).

This is a classic illustration of how an individual will project parts of themselves that they consider significant (sometimes unconsciously) onto an object that would otherwise have little meaning. This principle is central to creative expression and interventions.

Activity 4.1 can also be used in any session to quickly assess the mood and subject of participants. By asking for a "check-in" of feelings through magazine pictures (less time) or a painting (more time), personal experiences during the week can identify immediate, relevant, and significant themes.

## 4.2 Introductions #2

Social interaction.

### Objective

Introduction through questions and interaction.

### Implementation

1.  Form pairs and ask each other questions. There are many sides to each person. Don't ask about the obvious (name, school, work). Look for unusual details about each individual. Questions may be about favorite movie/foods/entertainer/place, "what are you frightened of?" "what is the funniest thing that has happened to you?" and "what would be your ideal job?" Learn as much about each other as possible in ten minutes.

2.  Each person introduces their partner to the group with the information they have learned and observation about emotions experienced/ demonstrated by either person in the conversation.

#### NOTE

The goal is not just to introduce each other. It is to detect in ten minutes how interesting that person is and introduce them to the group so that each member would like to know more about the person introduced. The increased disclosure is more likely to build genuine reciprocal interest and empathy.

Making an observation about the emotions of the activity partner relates to the skill of emotional decoding of self and other people.

## 4.3 Saying goodbye

Group appreciation, book.

In an open group, members usually come and go at different times. Group members will also become attached to staff members who may leave. When possible, give importance to a departure by making an announcement, expressing what was appreciated about the person and how much they will be missed. When a group itself finishes, a ritual such as the following can be introduced.

### Objective

Express appreciation, take positive reinforcement away from group.

## Implementation

1.   Using a template (pages for a book, petals of a flower, die cut shapes) give each group member a number of cardstock shapes – one for each other member of the group. Comments of appreciation are written on the card shapes, one for each person.

2.   When comments have been completed, each group member is given what others have written and appreciated about them. As a collection this provides an ongoing reminder of relationships built. It also expresses a range of positive behaviors and character traits that the individual may not have been aware was appreciated by others. The pieces can be kept together in a simple card or book-making exercise ("Books, journals, and cards," Chapter 8).

# CHAPTER 5

# Conceptual and cognitive processing

## Semantic and pragmatic weaknesses

This chapter's activities address differences in cognitive processing, prioritizing, and planning. Ideally, the early introduction of brainstorming and organization planning can be integrated into subsequent art/creative activities. Given the number and variety of intelligent and creative initiatives that have sprung from minds of people like Temple Grandin, Albert Einstein, Charles Darwin, and Thomas Jefferson, all of whom had AS traits (Ledgin 2002), the conclusion must be drawn that there is no lack of intelligence, but some difficulty in utilizing, processing, and expressing that intelligence.

Individuals with AS are typically curtailed by inflexible use of language – rules are rules, words are taken literally, and the larger picture can be lost in a sea of detail and facts. Yet our understanding of the world is a result of language and perceptions. Our choices – to vote, to buy a car, to respond to a friend – rely on our perceptions which are a product of what we have seen and heard. Bad decision making is likely if we have not gathered enough information because our information gives us a skewed impression of "the truth" or we have misunderstood the information. It is impossible, of course, to have all the information all the time. The extent and depth of our knowledge rests largely on our experience, our language (to acquire and understand information) and processing skills (to determine relevant information and its potential). If we can support decisions with reliable information that has come from different sources and different points of view (not simply our own experience), decisions will be more realistic and adaptable.

For a person who typically has concrete and literal thinking, the idea that there is not one truth or absolute answer to everything can be unsettling.

Learning to ask different questions and accept the validity of a variety of perspectives will open up whole new worlds. This is a skill needed at school to acquire information and interpret what is read and heard. It is a skill needed to make positive choices as an independent adult.

## Opening new doors

Asking a question that requires an answer in 30 words or less implies that there is one truth, easily articulated. In fact there is rarely one truth or right answer. A strategy of lateral thinking is to broaden perceptions, see the same thing from different perspectives and to look for richer, broader, more comprehensive answers. Traditional thinking systems are based on language rather than how the brain works (de Bono 1990). While useful for simplifying and forming self-organizing systems, language may actually prevent development of a richer code of communication and understanding with which to perceive experiences and information.

People with Asperger's Syndrome cannot rely on an easy use of language. The positive side to this is that the nonconventional thinking system of individuals with Asperger's Syndrome is rich in potential. Forcing their thoughts through a narrow channel of a few words is challenging and frustrating. It can choke off creative potential. The work of parents and professionals may be to find constructive, generative ways for creative thoughts and potential to be expressed.

Finally, the following activities tap into non-verbal, lateral, and creative open-ended strategies for thinking and retaining information. Activities should be modified and gradated according to skill level. Every opportunity should be given for physical and cognitive processes to reinforce each other. Individualize activities as much as possible – practice in groups will ideally be generalized to real life.

## Associative thinking: mind spiders and different perceptions

One of the oldest, simplest yet most effective tools for learning and organizing information is through images. Caveman drew on rocks – drawings which communicate with modern man. An image gives life to an abstract idea before words can be found for it. Images that suggest possibilities and precede organization are seen in the work of architects, dressmakers, and probably Santa's helpers. A picture is worth a thousand words. Combining pictures and words is an ideal way to stimulate original ideas and optimize processing of those ideas: the images suggest the words; the words bring intellect to the pictures. Many strategies have been used to stimulate and apply the creative process through images and words. Effective tools to use images to stimulate associations include the mind chart (MacGregor 1994) and mind map (de Bono 1993), flow charts and organizational trees.

One young man with AS who effectively uses the image association strategy describes it as "spider mind" or "spider map." Spider mind can be as simple or complex as desired. It displaces linear thinking with multidimensional thinking and allows the interplay of images and words. It utilizes colors, senses, and different perspectives to make associations and is easy and enjoyable.

Thinking of "work," people without strong AS traits typically recall a generalized idea. The idea of "work" might represent lifelong routine, reward, a variety of occupations. For the AS individual, "work" is more likely to recall a specific picture of their experience of work – perhaps Dad going to the office or chopping wood. Developing ideas and recalling information are usually limited to the situation-specific or experiential method of processing.

The spider mind begins with a central visual idea and radiates outward with an infinite number of associations – leaves on a branch, branches on a tree. Each of the associations has potential to be the center of another map of association. Associations are limited only by restraints of time and interest. A mind map provides a tool to extend a simplistic definition and to look at endless perspectives and associations. It begins with associations of pictures to be made between memories and senses (work: digging trenches, people in noisy trains, air-conditioned offices, leather bags, tools, smell of oil, books). Associations are infinite with each picture providing new potential. Yet the visual mapping provides a cohesiveness: connections and generalizations can be made (such as physical labor vs. mental work) and patterns identified.

Variations of this exercise, informally and formally, expand thinking beyond the obvious, the literal, and the experienced. Once group members become familiar with it, it can be integrated into activities in simpler versions and practiced as a natural approach to a problem or issue. It not only facilitates creative thought, but can also be an effective form of communication of ideas to other people. It offers an ideal hypothetical space to question the validity of "thinking trap" assumptions (jumping to conclusions, tunnel vision, all-or-nothing thinking, personalizing, externalizing, overgeneralizing, and emotional reasoning).

## 5.1 Spider mind: work

Collage, expressive art.

### Objective

To identify associative and recall possibilities of thinking in images and associations. Exploration of "work."

### Implementation

1. *What does the word "work" mean to you?* (Give a couple of minutes for a response, waiting until the answers have been exhausted.)

2. Provide a large sheet of paper and many different colored pens. In the center, draw a picture of what comes to mind with the word "work"; use different colors. From the central image, draw more than five non-straight lines toward the edges of the paper. Each line leads to an image associated with "work" – Money? Routine? Friends? representing a different image that the idea of "work" brings to mind. In a group, even at this early stage, different and very unique associations will be made, testament to the wonderful uniqueness and creativity of us all if we are not restricted to simplistic definitions created by other people.

3. Spend one minute on each of the ten images, beginning a series of ten associations for each of them (that's 100 if you complete them): include words but only after the images – let the images define the words, not the words define the images. Even the connecting lines can be thick, thin, curved, suggestive. Use colors in the associations (suggestive and easier recall) and continue to let all of the senses play a part in the associations – this is an exercise of the senses more than of the intellect. Be spontaneous, integrate memories, surreal images, anything and everything that springs from the mind now that the creative gate has been opened.

4. Repeat the first step of the exercise: *What does the word "work" mean to you?* Now the descriptions are less likely to be a dry collection of precise words and memories; and more imaginative, innovative, comprehensive, expansive, expressive. Most of all, the description of career is likely to be enthusiastic and the participant is personally engaged – all sorts of possibilities remain unexplored and the mind is yearning to finish what it has started – an impossible, challenging, and satisfying task (and fitting the criteria of Mihaly Csikszentmihalyi's (1990) "flow" experience).

The information is also easy to summarize and recall because of the visual and associative components. Information is chunked into relevant groups and flows with an organic, individualized momentum toward countless potentially generative possibilities. "Work" is no longer bound by experience and language but is a dynamic concept. Pictures leave concepts open to be interpreted and reinterpreted from different perspectives, not confining them forever to a few words. A mind map is easy to review and can be added to over time, with more information, insights, maturity, experience – all integrated without disrupting the order characteristic of a linear "one-answer" approach.

This exercise can be done regularly with different concepts – the more often it is practiced the more natural it will become. It is an excellent problem-solving tool. A theme that is personalized allows endless possibilities for internal and external perceptions to be realized and ability to be authentic in the response. Here is another theme to explore.

## 5.2 Spider mind: transitions

Mind map, collage, expressive art.

### Objective

Identify experiences, feelings, and potential problems associated with transitions.

### Implementation

1. Do a spider map on problems and feelings that you have experienced during a change or transition in your life. Example: moving school or house. What were the good and the bad outcomes of the change?

2. Take branches of the map into the future. What changes and transitions can you expect in the future? What associated problems may there be?

3. Using this information, explore possible solutions to the problems. What can you do now to lessen difficulties that may arise from changes in the future?

4. Identify the feelings you have about possible changes in the future. (How will you feel if you have to leave all of your friends at this school and move to another state?) If you can't do anything to lessen difficulties (or identify all the difficulties), what changes can you make to your thoughts and feelings to make it a more positive experience? (What is there to look forward to in the move? What can you gain/get excited about?)

*Other suggested themes*

- Having Asperger's Syndrome
- School
- Career
- Family relationships
- Future goals
- Fear
- Concentration
- Imagination
- Intelligence
- Organization and self-discipline
- Initiative

Thematic ideas and words need not be complete. They can ask a question. Buzan and Buzan (1993), whose *Mind Map Book* is recommended for its comprehensive review and visual examples of mind maps, suggest the following:

- If I could…
- Buy a…
- Learn a…
- Change a…
- Withdraw from a…
- Begin a…
- Create a…

Creative activities: spider maps, spider minds, mind maps, and mapping are very useful tools for developing a collage or any form of art, on any theme.

> **Ingenuity/originality/practical intelligence/street smarts**
> Some of the strengths that enhance resilience are original thought, practical intelligence, and ability to problem solve. Spider maps and other visual and/or alternative, non-linear ways of processing facilitate them.

## Different caps: different perspectives

Another author who makes significant contributions to alternative ways of thinking and processing is Edward de Bono. Just as a technique of Gestalt therapy is the "empty chair technique" (imagine the "smart me" sitting there – what would he say?), de Bono suggests wearing different hats ("putting on our thinking caps") to introduce different perspectives or perceptions (imagine you're wearing the red hat – what are your feelings about the subject?). The "Six Thinking Hats" technique is elaborated on in de Bono's book *Teaching Children to Think* (1993), which contains many excellent games and exercises to develop cognitive processing skills with lateral and critical "broad and detailed" thinking. The following props and symbols can be used to represent different perspectives:

- chairs
- hats
- puppets
- cut-out cardstock shapes (hearts, magic wands)
- a variety of props – keys (giving freedom), rocks (to suggest weight being carried), microphone (giving power to be heard and understood).

Perspectives suggested by these cues or props might include:

- feelings about the subject (sitting in the red chair, identify angry feelings about school; sitting in the green chair, identify the happy feelings about school)
- perspective of consequences (wearing the red hat, identify the negative consequences of going to college; wearing the green hat, identify the positive consequences of going to college)
- different possible outcomes (through the "optimistic smiling puppet," identify the best possible outcome; through the "cranky pessimistic puppet," identify the worst possible outcome)
- way-out wacky alternatives (using a magic wand, conjure up magical alternatives and outcomes)
- weak links in the chain – why something may not work, possible problems (a broken chain); why it might work anyway (a bottle of glue)
- a Martian's perception (a Martian puppet)

- perspective of instinct, gut feelings, and inner tuition
- perspective of what it would take – realistic checklist, perhaps with other people's input.

## 5.3 Making decisions about a vacation

Props, puppets.

### Objective

Look at an issue from different perspectives. In reaching a decision there can be many valid arguments and perspectives. Cooperate and compromise in bringing different perspectives together for application of a decision that satisfies as many people as possible. Check for "thinking traps" (jumping to conclusions, tunnel vision, all-or-nothing thinking, personalizing, externalizing, overgeneralizing, and emotional reasoning).

### Implementation

1.    Give a different perspective to each prop or puppet (e.g. a label or sign around their neck). Allocate a different puppet/perspective to each person. Perspectives can be chosen for group members or they can choose their own. Examples: an old person puppet; a sporty puppet; a stay-at-home puppet.

2.    Improvise a conversation between the puppets as the theme is discussed. Each puppet takes a turn in proposing its perspective, to which each other puppet is given the opportunity to put its interpretation on that perspective from its own perspective.

3.    Other puppets can also question the validity of "thinking trap" behavior (jumping to conclusions, tunnel vision, all-or-nothing thinking, personalizing, externalizing, overgeneralizing, and emotional reasoning). Examples: It always rains when I go to the beach. There's nothing for Grandpas to do on a vacation. Questioning other people's views should be done in a cooperative, non-confrontational manner.

4.    Make a game of suggesting unusual compromises. (Perhaps the less adventurous person can drive the boat while his grandchildren water-ski.)

5.    An observer can make notes of suggestions to be discussed later. The information is compared, balanced, prioritized, and compromises reached.

6.   A variation on this exercise is to integrate it with a spider map – different perceptions, different branches and associations. The difference with this activity is to integrate different perspectives for a single course of action.

## Goals and organization

*Recalling specific facts*

With adolescence, many individuals seem to be coping far better than they were as youngsters. They have modeled their behavior and learned, one way or another, what is expected of them. But there are still underlying differences in ways of thinking and learning, causing difficulties that may not be obvious. An inclination to be messy and untidy might be exacerbated by an inability to organize things and thoughts. It should not be taken for granted that the AS individual can organize themselves.

Education increasingly requires an ability to recall and present relevant information in a concise and cohesive manner (for example, write a 300-word essay on the grape industry in Europe). It is no longer enough to be able to recall a string of facts. Information now has to be understood and written about in a wider context, a bigger picture, with associations and implications. The AS individual may have difficulties with the overall conceptual picture.

### SORTING OUT THE INFORMATION

From the central theme (title of essay, assignment, theme) break relevant information into chunks. Simplify the essence, don't get lost in details. Make an art out of detecting and highlighting key words or phrases that encompass the essence of an argument. When making notes of a lecture or reading a text, don't just learn the facts. Identify an outline or structure. Take slabs of associated information with a common thread and "box" it. Identify causes and effects, consequences, and conceptual vs. descriptive information. Give information a place on a cohesive visual map, with hooks for easier recall through association or visual cues.

### MEMORY HOOKS

As an example, if structuring information about the grape industry in Europe, the first section might be "hooked" with a key word ("history"), a picture ("monk in the Dark Ages"), or a position on a structure (timeline). Each slab of information is both broken into smaller sections and given a position in a larger pattern. Synonyms can be used to retrieve information verbally, pictures to retain and retrieve information visually.

Facts can be fitted to a structure like a spider map with associations numbered for appropriate sequencing in a linear presentation. An example was made earlier of a student fitting information to a cohesive whole by hanging different parts to the shape of a tree – main arguments and peripheral arguments. Details should be "chunked" into one area. The scenario can be as complicated as required, and generally the more absurd the visual associations, the more easily recalled. Other organizing strategies for studying include story maps, topic mapping and webbing (Fullerton *et al.* 1996). These provide basic structures for main points to be arranged and connected with lines, drawn either in preparation of a class or while the class is being taught.

For better organization, study habits should be structured. Compartmentalize time and space. Break available time into sections, structure and prioritize activities accordingly. For example, at the beginning of a semester, allocate time for specific projects. If 30 pages of facts can be absorbed in a day, don't leave two days for reading a textbook of 200 pages. Break it up and allow time for reviewing. If it takes two weeks to finish an assignment, block that time out in a planner. Structure time and plan expenditure of energy.

When time is planned, take into consideration optimum times for study during the day. Is it better to study in the morning or night? Is there a place that makes it easier to study (a library, the desk in the bedroom)? Are there some things needed to study efficiently (quiet, not hungry)? Allow for time to relax and review.

Keep study notes, assignment sheets, and relevant paperwork, pens, calculator, and tools organized. Keep small things in a box that can be carried easily from one place to another. Use different folders and files for different subjects. Checklist things to be done. Each subject should have a planning chart of tasks to be completed, due dates for assignments, and a timeline. (Does material have to be collected or task completed before a particular assignment can be done?) Draw graphic charts to illustrate organization plans and details clearly.

Keep one diary or calendar for time management and a list of things to do. In that, priorities can be noted with references to projects detailed in the subject folders. Keep the diary or calendar itself organized, easy to read, perhaps color coded. Use it as an overview and reminder. Be in the habit of carrying it for reference, making new notes, and checking on the list of things to do.

Regularly reorganize paperwork. Ann Fullerton *et al.* (1996) suggest that paper management can be broken down into three basic steps:

- Throw it away.
- Act on it.
- File it.

A reminder card with words to this effect can be kept pinned on a desk as a visual cue to make a habit of organization.

> **Judgment/critical thinking/open-mindedness**
> Strengths that enhance resilience include the ability to assess situations, make appropriate judgments, think critically, and have an open mind.

Organization of information and life requires judgment and critical thinking. In order to achieve the simplest goal, there has to be an overall view of the process toward a desired outcome. Being organized in one area does not easily generalize to organization in new or unfamiliar areas for someone with AS traits. The Three-Step Plan described below provides a structure to categorize and simplify steps in novel situations. An important principle is to consider the link between choices of action and potential consequences before a decision is made.

After the introduction, the Three-Step Plan can be practiced in two activities: Plan a party (5.5) and Budget and money goals (5.6). While tedious at first, practice should make the principles more easily understood and integrated.

## 5.4 Three-Step Plan: facts, exploration, action

Organizational device.

### Objective

Categorize steps of organization for decision making and action. There is more than one way of seeing and doing something – assess, think critically, make appropriate judgments.

### Implementation

1. *Collect facts*: The desired outcome, the reasons and motivation, the circumstances, the resources.

2.    *Explore possibilities, options*: Explore possibilities, alternatives, options, consequences, risks, possible solutions to potential problems, in order to make an educated guess on the best course of action. What would be possible consequences of different decisions? This is an ideal step to use creative and associative thinking – novel ways of putting together the known elements. Consider other people's perspectives. Take note of feelings. Emotions and motivation are interlinked. The planning is more crucial than the execution.

3.    *Reality check, decision making, organization*: With the known facts and information about potential directions and choices, make a decision. Identify concrete steps necessary to reach the goal, sequenced appropriately; costs, compromises, and possible weak links identified (remember, a chain is only as strong as its weakest link). What preparations can be made before execution of the plan to strengthen weak links or prevent problems?

## 5.5 Plan a party

Three-Step Plan, mind map.

### Objective

Plan a party using alternative ways of processing (mind maps, thinking caps) with the Three-Step Plan.

### Implementation

Use the Three-Step Plan above and one or a combination of the above creative brainstorming techniques, to explore the possibilities for a party.

1.    Collect facts. When, where, why have a party. Limitations (space, parents, budget, time). Who would be invited.

2.    Use creative and associative thinking to develop possibilities, alternatives, options, consequences, risks. What are different party themes, variations on location, time, food, music. What are the potential consequences of these options? List the costs, possible difficulties, and creative solutions. Even in a logical exercise such as this, feelings play an important role. For example, if there are feelings of anxiety, what is the cause and what are ways of dealing with it?

3.    Action. With information from the previous step, what are the best decisions and choices? Convert this information back into concrete

steps, prioritized and sequenced. Organize a timeline (times to send invitations, shop for food, etc.).

## 5.6 Budget and money goals

Three-Step Plan, mind map.

### Objective

Organize budget and money goals using alternative ways of processing – spider maps, thinking caps, etc. – with the Three-Step Plan.

### Implementation

Use the Three-Step Plan and one or a combination of the above creative techniques to do a personal budget. Instructions should be paraphrased to suit individual levels of skill and circumstances.

1. Collect facts (what you have, don't have); reasons and motivation for a budget; what the goal is; circumstances; resources.

2. Explore possibilities, ambitions, options, and potential in making and saving money, possible modifications in areas where money is spent, potential problems in reaching the money goal. What are the potential consequences of different options? How do you feel about making and saving money? Identify feelings as you explore different aspects of this exercise. Emotions will sustain or inhibit motivation. What can you do to increase emotions that will support motivation? (Perhaps visualization of what can be done with the money.) Use creative and associative thinking.

3. Using information from the previous step, what are the best decisions and choices? Convert this information back into a budget – concrete, prioritized, and sequenced. When looking at the concrete plan, what possible weak links are there? What preparations can be made to strengthen the weak links or prevent problems?

As with the visual brainstorming maps, integrate the Three-Step Plan to problem solving as a matter of course as often as possible. With practice and familiarity, it will be more easily generalized to real-life situations.

The following exercises elaborate on the third step of the Three-Step Plan – *organization*. The facts are clear (for example, toothache) and the options for action are limited (let the toothache get worse or go to a dentist). For low-functioning individuals who have difficulty to the extent that it impacts on self-care, the third step, organization and execution of the plan, can be immobilizing. The third step ("action") can be broken down further to help sequencing of the necessary steps. Visual maps such as cartoons are helpful. Support cartoons for specific scenarios can be constructed with the help of a parent or professional.

## 5.7 Self-organization

Cartoon, film strip, role play, letter writing.

These help break down big sequences into smaller steps and mental rehearsal. They are visual cues for carrying out the steps and can be kept as a reminder for future situations.

### Objective

Locate a professional: visual map sequences for organizing specific tasks.

### Implementation

1.  Identify a task likely to arise in the course of everyday life (for example, need to visit a dentist).

2.  Draw a cartoon (might just be faces with voice balloons) with the following steps or film strip. Craft shops and scrapbook supply stores sell die cuts of a film strip, or a template can be made to suggest a film strip. As each frame of the film strip is finished, the subject matter can be elaborated upon through questions, discussion, or relevant activities.

3.  *First frame of film strip/cartoon. Theme: Can family or friends help?*
    If there is pain in the mouth, in the teeth, who is a family member who could give advice? Draw a frame of speaking to that family member and telling them about the problem. Have they had this problem? Can they recommend someone who fixed the problem?

4.  *Second frame. Theme: Finding professional help.*
    If a family member can't help you, find phone numbers for people working in that profession in the local telephone directory. Look up numbers and study advertisements. Who is someone paid to help in this situation? Draw a frame of using the telephone book to find a professional.

5.  *Third frame. Theme: Contacting professional.*
    Telephone the office of the professional person. Speak to the person who answers the phone. Role play making telephone calls: Ask questions

(explain the problem – important information without unnecessary detail). Can they help? When can the doctor/dentist see you? How much will it cost and/or what should you bring? Make an appointment. Ask for the address and details about how to get to the address. Write details in your appointment book/personal diary. Draw a frame of being on the telephone, asking questions, and making an appointment.

6. *Fourth frame. Theme: Visiting professional #1.*
When the time comes to visit the professional, get there five or ten minutes early. There may be paperwork to fill out. If necessary, ask the secretary or person at the desk to help you with the paperwork. (Always get a receipt for money you have paid, and put it in a "personal finances file" at home.) Draw a frame of being in the office, speaking to the secretary.

7. *Fifth frame. Theme: Visiting professional #2.*
When you speak to the doctor or professional, you should have a list of symptoms or questions you'd like to ask. This person is being paid to look after your problem. Be sure that he or she has all the information they need to help. If you are confused about anything, ask more questions or ask the professional to write it down for you to understand it better or remember it later. If there is medication to be taken, ask for detailed written instructions. Draw a frame of speaking with the professional, asking questions, making notes.

8. *Sixth frame. Theme: Satisfaction.*
If you are not happy with the work a professional has done, what can you do? If you went to the dentist and the problem has not been fixed or reoccurred within a short time, call the office of that professional again. Tell the secretary over the telephone that the problem has reoccurred. Make another appointment.

   If you have seen the professional to fix the problem and not been happy with the results, if you have visited again and the problem has still not been fixed, start the process again. Find another professional. Don't keep going back to someone if you don't feel comfortable with them, if you can't talk to them about your problem, or the problem is not being fixed. Just because someone's a "professional" or an expert doesn't mean they're right for you. Sometimes it is necessary to visit more than one person to find someone who you feel good about and works well with you.

9. If you are confused, look for a friendly person (preferably someone who works in the office) and ask them for help: "Could you help me please?" If someone has been friendly and helpful to you, thank them. Ask them their name and use it. Remember their name in case you are in the office again. If someone has been particularly helpful over a period of time,

write them a simple thank you note: "Dear Mrs... Thank you for the help you gave me with my... It was appreciated very much. Sincerely, Chris Smith."

10. Keep receipts and paperwork from professional visits. Why is organization important? What is likely to happen if you aren't organized?

11. The film strip can be enacted and videotaped for reinforcing the steps.

## Motor coordination

Difficulties with fine and gross motor skills, clumsiness, and lack of coordination are common AS traits. This book is simply to introduce concepts that contribute to resilient development and some activities that can be easily integrated into a generalized support program. For more comprehensive support of fine and motor skill difficulties, occupational therapy is recommended.

### Metronome activities

A lack of motor coordination is most apparent in physical awkwardness but has also been associated with lack of attention, cognitive processing, speech, reading skills, and self-regulation of emotion. Motor coordination, focus, attention, and control can be improved through practice of coordination of simple physical activities with rhythm (Schaffer *et al.* 2001). The rhythm can be established with a metronome or ticking clock. Some sophisticated apparatus has been developed to finely tune individual response to increased periods of time and levels of concentration. The following activities are more basic but demonstrate application of the same principles. Use a metronome to establish a rhythm. Following the rhythm as precisely as possible:

- tap a foot
- clap hands
- tap foot while clapping hands
- alternate clapping own hands and then giving "high fives" with a partner
- vary simple activities to coordinate with beat of the metronome – concentrate on precision, increasing lengths of time.

## 5.8 Leisure activities and motor skills

Physical exercise.

### Objective

Find an enjoyable activity to practice motor skills, grace, agility, physical control, rhythm. Tai Chi and yoga are helpful for relaxation and mood regulation. Basic yoga activities are introduced in Chapter 6. Forty minutes of physical exercise can reduce stress levels for two or three hours.

### Implementation

Ask a local practitioner to demonstrate and do a session with group members on one or more of the following. It is useful in itself but might also initiate an interest to be developed outside of the support group.

- Aikido (non-violent martial art)
- Tai Chi
- Yoga.

## High–low: fast–slow

Thanks to Benjamin Boone (1989) for suggesting variations on movement/ music/singing exercises to add the dimensions of pitch and body–space relationships:

> Have group members start by sitting on the floor. With any instrument, play in the mid-range and tell them that when you play HIGHER, to gradually stand, and when you play LOWER, to get closer to the floor (demonstrate, using high and low pitches). Begin playing, using a consistently rising or falling contour. As they get used to this game, you can execute more complex contours (i.e., go up a little, then back down, go up a little more, then back down, then way up high, then way low, etc.). This simple game ingrains pitch contour recognition. FAST–SLOW can be added for interest and fun.

## Movement

Movement and free dance introduce a variety of activities that can be designed to suit the individual. First, it can be used as physical exercise and a leisure activity. Second, the movement and free dance activities offer a variety of opportunities to strengthen traits that may cause difficulty such as motor coordination and balance; interaction and spatial relationships with other people and objects; and emotional expression (Figure 5.1).

Stretching and warming up is an important part of a movement activity. It can become an important activity in itself, being modeled by a leader, or improvised to match the mood of music or percussion. Forming a circle, moving around it, or weaving in and out of it can set up a coordinated and rhythmic movement with others, and require awareness of each other's space.

One of the most important factors in building resilience is to make meaningful connections, including connections to one's own culture. If there are cultural differences in a group, develop activities from this. Encourage each member to tell stories about their cultural background, perhaps introducing a folk story or bringing typical food to snack time. Introducing props, music, and dance that are culture specific not only reinforces cultural identity but makes connections with other group members who might enjoy the activity. Local social and culture clubs may have members who are willing to provide music and give a culture-specific dance lesson to the group. Below is a sample lesson, using Zorba's Dance, from *Freedom to Move* by Dunphy and Scott (2003, p.108).

## 5.9 Moving together

Folk dance, music, movement.

### Objective

To move as part of a large group.

> Folk dance offers experiences of different movement patterns. Dancing together as part of a large group offers opportunities for leadership and co-operation and experiences of new patterns and directions for moving through space. This can be both enjoyable and a challenge, especially for those people who find co-operation and physical contact difficult. One dance we have enjoyed offers all of these experiences.
>
> Zorba's Dance – dancing anti-clockwise in shoulder hold
>
> The infamous Zorba's Dance, a popular form of the traditional Greek syrtaki, is danced in a semi-circle, with dancers connected in a shoulder hold. This positioning contrasts with the holds of the set dance of the Anglo-Celtic traditions, which requires people to physically connect only by an occasional touch of hand or elbows. Travel patterns are different too. In Greek circle dances, participants always move anti-clock-

wise, following the leadership of the person at the head of the line, while in set dances, travel patterns are mostly forward and backward steps.

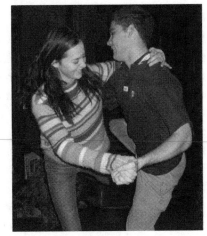

*Starting position*
Dancers stand in a line with arms in shoulder hold (i.e. arms laid along the neighbor's upper arms). Leader stands on far right end of the line.

FOOTWORK: Three steps travelling anti-clockwise (R, L, R) and lift L leg; step to left on L and lift R leg; repeat throughout the music. This step speeds up and slows down with the music.

*Figure 5.1 Movement*

DIRECTION OF TRAVEL: Dance travels anti-clockwise.

FACING DIRECTION: Dancers face into center of circle.

*Variations*
*Simple version*
Step on R, L, R, pause; step on L, pause; repeat.

HOLD: instead of shoulder hold, dancers connect by holding hands.

*Complex version*
PATTERNS: the leader can make even simple steps interesting by leading the group all around the space, varying direction and travel pattern.

FINISH POSITION: The leader brings group to make small circle, all facing in.

MUSIC TRADITIONAL VERSION: soundtrack, Zorba the Greek. Disco version: LCD (1998) Zorba's Dance.

Other music suggested by Kim Dunphy and Jenny Scott is in Appendix 2. It is categorized according to mood – dreamy, dramatic, playful, "otherworldly," energetic – and can be used for relaxation, dance, movement, art, and background mood.

## Music therapy

Music can be introduced in a variety of ways, and tailored to meet individual needs. Its versatility is discussed here, to be considered and perhaps integrated with other activities for cognitive processing, self-awareness, and social interaction. More specific musical activities are suggested later in the book.

Music is a tool that supports conventional teaching objectives. One program of psychodynamic music therapy for younger children on the autistic spectrum integrated the principles of structure and schedules of Division TEACCH (Treatment and Education of Autistic and related Communication handicapped CHildren) and was assessed by Ruth Walsh-Stewart (2002).

The objective was to use music to improve social skills and emotional communication. Implementation employed boundaries, visual cues, and specific songs to satisfy the structured learning principles of TEACCH. The musical component of the workshops allowed individual freedom to choose and play instruments, and the degree and improvisation of participation.

The results of a ten-week group revealed a general improvement in "attention, social skills, and musical response." More specifically, for at least one child (on whom the study focused), there was increased attention over time and interaction with the group facilitator, increased sensitivity to mood and rhythm, playing music cooperatively with other group members, both leading and following, and increased creativity. The study suggests that variations on "making music together" can be used regularly as warm-up activities, to encourage participation or evoke emotion, to promote group cohesion and cooperation with facilitator and other group members. As familiarity is welcomed by most AS individuals, this might be an appropriate opening or closing ritual each week.

John Ortiz writes of integrating music in many ways in *The Tao of Music* (1997). This book also contains exercises and extensive music suggestions. Just as behavior, thoughts, and emotions interact to impact on our lives, music can impact on our behavior thoughts and emotions, and consequently our lives. For example, in the case of depression, energizing music can stimulate physical effort and enthusiasm; accompanying music or making sounds through singing, humming, or instruments can help express feelings and emotions; music can change moods, perceptions, and thoughts. Given these multimodal effects, music can be manipulated to support deliberate efforts to make changes. Creative activities can be designed to integrate music (such as a background of recorded music) or designed to focus on the music itself (making sounds through voice and instruments).

## Designing activities with music

As the TEACCH study above revealed, simply playing musical instruments in a group can improve "attention, social skills, and musical response." However, just as good-quality art materials are likely to evoke a better experience, good-quality instruments are likely to be more exciting to the participant.

Positive affirmations and visualizations can be stimulated and supported by music – effective in a variety of activities from relaxation and goal setting to "letting go" of issues. It can reduce stress and anxiety and be an effective relaxation tool, triggering endorphins. Meditative music can be used to help regulate and control breathing, facilitating exercises in self-control and regulation, thought stopping, focusing, and "centering" (Ortiz 1997). Centering involves listening to the body, increasing consciousness of feelings and reactions – "focus on what your heart, body and mind are telling you."

Rhythmic synchronicity and ways of increasing it is discussed in Chapter 7. Ortiz suggests that anger has its own rhythm and listening to a well-chosen piece of music, and "getting in sync" with it, will effectively reduce the feelings of anger. Rhythm set by background music can also set a tempo for organization and tasks, while it energizes and increases positive mood. Socially, background music has been shown to significantly increase the positive feelings people have toward each other. Group members and facilitators are likely to respond more positively to each other if there is background music (baroque, strings, melodious music). At the same time, be aware that some individuals may be supersensitive to extra noise in their environment – be sensitive to unique responses to the same music.

While professional music therapists and many good books on the subject can offer more comprehensive information for AS groups, music can easily be applied in nearly every setting and every group in some way to effectively complement a program for individuals with Asperger's Syndrome.

## Collaborative poetry

Poetry offers a marvelous opportunity to express and validate a unique, often emotional, way of thinking and looking at the world. Response to a theme can circumvent conventional and literal use of language, using analogy or words to describe surreal or visual images and connections.

Writing poetry collaboratively can be an inspiring and high-spirited group activity, and encourage individual efforts. Each person might write a line on a theme or words can be written for them if the task of writing is laborious and inhibits inspiration. The written lines are then shuffled and reorganized as a poem. Students are likely to have fun playing against each other with words, outdoing each other while elaborating on a theme.

Rhyming is not as important as expression of ideas. Unity can be achieved through each line beginning with the same words ("I wish," "If I could sing…," "when I am King…."). Another uniting "rule" could be to use a sense in each line (taste, touch, etc.) or a metaphor (symbolic thinking). Kenneth Koch (1970) has written a very helpful book called *Wishes, Lies, and Dreams* which gives more detail on teaching children to write poetry. He writes that a popular theme with children is "I used to…but now…," documenting changes in the way the individual acts and thinks.

## Playing with words

Individuals with AS typically enjoy words and can be a little pedantic about how they are used. Unfortunately, words may also be a source of confusion and frustration when other people aren't as literal or careful about their use. A big issue in relationships is the tendency to be literal in conversation. Many AS individuals find themselves in difficulties because they tend to take things literally – and relationships generally require a certain amount of forgiveness and leniency to survive. The following exercise is "playing" with words.

## 5.10 Word games

Language use.

### Objective

Identify, understand, and use non-literal language appropriately.

### Implementation

1.  Provide a handout defining, comparing, and giving examples of the following:

    *   Hyperbole – strong exaggeration: He is the best sailor in the whole world!

    *   Simile – using comparative words: The sea is *like* glass.

    *   Metaphor – equates objects: The sea *is* glass.

    *   Personification – giving human qualities: It's an angry sea.

    *   Symbol – represents a concept: The sea of life.

    *   Teasing and sarcasm: Tom, sailor in the desert.

NOTE
The difference between teasing and the negativity embedded in sarcasm may be detected by tone of voice or facial expression. Sarcasm is not normally complimentary but denigrating. Some people find sarcasm funny (as in "roasts"), but because it is also used as an insult it can be misused or misunderstood. When someone else uses sarcasm, their underlying motivation or agenda might be questioned.

2.    Take turns to make up sentences that use hyperboles, similes, etc. Discuss in the group an appropriate context when they might be used.

3.    Take a phrase like "Tom the fish expert" that can be used with variations as both complimentary and as an insult and use facial expressions and tone to change the meaning or implication of the same phrase.

4.    Make a competition of collecting metaphors and similes. Examples: I was boiling mad. He works like a horse. She really cracks me up.

## 5.11 More word games

Language use.

It can be difficult for people with Asperger's Syndrome to hold four or five things in their working memory at once, or to organize and retrieve a sequence of information in their heads. As with most things, practice of this skill may not cure but can only improve it. Take five minutes on a car trip or traveling on a bus, with a friend or alone, to play games that practice accumulating information and being able to recall it either in order or a particular format.

### Objective
Practice memory retrieval.

### Implementation
The most basic game is "I went shopping and I bought...," gradually adding items to the list, retrieving the list each time, before adding another item. Variations might include:

• names of teams

• boys' names/girls' names

• occupations

• cities of the world.

Memory and mental organization:

1. Name six (or eight or ten) cities (or animals, television shows, song titles).

2. List them in order of length of name, from shortest to longest.

3. List them in order of length of name, from longest to shortest.

4. List them in order of how appealing they are to you.

5. List them in alphabetical order.

6. Alternate the list of cities with the list of animals (television shows, song titles) in alphabetical order.

7. Invent a new game that requires retrieval and organization.

8. Add rhyming words, words with the same number of syllables, and so on, increasing difficulty with level of skill. Ask individuals to invent their own memory games.

## 5.12 Generalize, categorize, discriminate

Word games.

It is important to be able to think in terms of categories and to be able to identify where something fits into a pattern or a bigger picture.

### Objective

Practice taking information and seeing it in terms of how it fits into a bigger picture and may be part of a greater whole, through categorization or generalization.

### Implementation

ACTIVITY #I

1. Each person brings a leaf from outside into the classroom. Each leaf is complete on its own and in its own way different from other leaves. Yet they have many things in common. Each leaf is part of a bigger tree, part of a bigger picture or pattern of information.

2. What do the leaves have in common and what information can we gain from looking at the similarities? (Do the leaves come from the same tree? Is there anything to indicate the time of season through looking at the leaves in a group? Do they have similar shapes or size or color?)

3. What differences are there and what information can we gain from looking at the differences? (Do they come from different trees? Are they different colors? Do different species have different qualities?)

ACTIVITY #2

1.   Take a group of magazine pictures and sort them according to dominant color, medium (drawing, photography), and "mood." Does a picture suggest happiness, sadness, emptiness? Categorize them accordingly.

2.   Discuss and discriminate – what are the features that determine how a group can be categorized? (What makes a "sad" picture sad?) In that particular group of pictures, how many different categories can be made through focusing on some feature or detail? (Example, people vs. objects; old vs. new.)

ACTIVITY #3

1.   Each person is like a leaf on a tree. They are different but there are similarities as well. They are individuals but they share communities and categories.

2.   Discuss in a group how you have things in common with other people and how you are different. Each person can take a different colored marker (Susan red; Ben blue) and write their names on small pieces of paper or card. Categorize names in relevant piles:

   •   Asian, European, African American.

   •   Usually talkative, usually quiet.

   •   Likes sport, doesn't like physical activities much.

   •   Plays a musical instrument, doesn't play a musical instrument.

   Note how everybody has some things in common but nobody is just like us. How can we use this information? Amongst other things, we can't assume other people think like us or react like us to the same things. Nor can we assume that they don't share at least some of our thoughts and feelings. People who look or seem different may have many things in common with us.

Activity 5.12 can be extended to introduce the theme of outward appearance. Style of dress and grooming make an impression on other people about the sort of person we are. Typically, outward appearance is not important to the AS individual and they don't recognize eccentricity in dress. Is the impression we make on other people important? When might it be important? How might people categorize us according to our dress? What sort of impression do we want to make in different circumstances? How can we change different features in our image and the way we present ourselves to change the impression we give other people?

## 5.13 Priorities

Prioritizing information.

When pieces of information are not seen as part of a bigger picture, it is difficult to gauge their importance and prioritize them. What is urgent in one situation may lose its importance in another situation. Being able to establish priorities is a key to organization.

### Objective

Prioritize information. Discern levels of importance and the difference between "desired" and "needed."

### Implementation

1. You wake up on a Saturday morning, walk into the kitchen and everybody is busy. Mom has to get your brother to his soccer game and asks you to feed the dog, put the breakfast dishes in the dishwasher, and get your dirty clothes ready to be washed by the time she gets back in an hour. Your baby sister is crying because she is hungry. Mom has put her cereal in her bowl but it is still sitting on the table and your sister can't reach it. Your father comes into the room and says, "For heaven's sake, turn that music down Ben – I can't hear myself think." This is going to be a very busy morning because you also have homework to do and you were going to telephone your friend Sean. You haven't even had breakfast yet.

2. Like a jigsaw puzzle, all of these things have to be made to fit into one frame: the time frame of today, Saturday, the time it takes from now until all of these things have been completed. Where do you start?

3. Write down everything that has to be done. Cut up the paper that the tasks are written on so that everything has its own piece of paper. Rearrange the pieces of paper so that each is given the correct priority. Accompany the finished list with a timeline – the time frame of today.

4. Of course, in real time no one will be appreciative of pieces of paper adding to the chaos of a busy Saturday morning. But use this exercise to discuss priorities and identify a system to quickly establish priorities. *What is desired? Needed? Urgent? Important? What's the difference?* In the following pairs, which should be given first priority and why?

   • The telephone rings just as something good comes up on television.

   • Your mom needs help in the kitchen – visitors are coming for lunch and she has to cook a meal for them. Your dad needs help cleaning up the yard. Who would you help and why?

- You see an accident and the person needs help. You are on your way to the shop for your mother – home is two minutes behind you and the shop is five minutes in front of you. What would you do and why?

Can group members think of dilemmas that may occur and need to be prioritized?

Although storytelling is a form of communication and perhaps should be included under social interaction in Chapter 7, the skills within storytelling include organization, mental sequencing, memory, and cohesiveness in the retelling so, for that reason, storytelling is included here.

## Narratives and storytelling

Encourage storytelling in all forms. Telling life stories practices articulation, staying "on track," being understood. Making up stories is even better. Imagination comes into play, along with mental images. Links and connections – sometimes not fully formulated or justified – are formed for a cohesive and sequenced flow of ideas. Encourage stories that express feelings and ideas rather than being purely descriptive (Figure 5.2).

Listening to others' stories and understanding their significance is important. Retelling stories encourages attentive listening skills and the ability to repeat the substance of a communication. Retelling a shorter version of a story, or summarizing it, requires discarding less important details while retaining the essence. Organization, pragmatics, and semantics will be enhanced.

Storytelling is a tool for illustrating how ideas and concepts can be applied to real life, symbolized in language, relating them to a larger picture that offers concrete connections. Storytelling is also an interesting way to learn. Information is more easily memorized and told from different perspectives and perceptions, including hypothetical situations, and storytelling can be fun for all ages. Storytelling can be practiced in a variety of creative ways: orally; visually – a journal, cartoons, expressive art; scriptwriting and drama; puppet shows. Here are a number of themes and ways of introducing a story:

## 5.14 Storytelling

Oral story.

### Objective

Encourage listening skills, practice articulation, express feelings and ideas.

### Implementation

1. Provide an ambiguous or cryptic picture and have a competition to see who can make up a most interesting/funny story about it. Credit or tokens can be given for originality, appropriate use of words, clarity, and "staying on track."

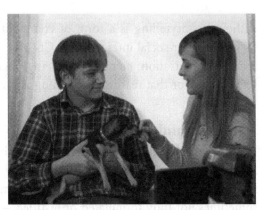

*Figure 5.2 Narratives and storytelling*

2. Suggest a theme such as "Stranded on Mars," "My sister the giraffe," or "The day my dreams came true" and ask for a picture to be painted. Then invite group members to make interpretations of their own work, along with a story about associated events, feelings, potential outcomes. Give credit for degree of cohesive elaboration, originality, attempts to express feelings or emotions, articulation, and so on. Discriminate between descriptive words and feeling words. Ask group members to tell a story in purely descriptive words, and then retell the story with feeling, expressive words.

3. Storytell a round by giving the first group member a sentence such as "It was a green and tingly day and I felt wonderful" or "I couldn't have imagined that would happen to me." Invite each group member to add a sentence or a few sentences to the evolving story, before passing the baton, so to speak, to the next person. A variation on this can be to throw a dice which calls group members (with pre-assigned numbers) to continue with the story with no particular order. This would encourage members to have an idea of where they might take the story if the dice puts them back in the "hot seat."

4. Introduce a subject which encourages the storyteller to project him or herself into the story. Young children might be asked what animal they would like to be and paint/tell a story about that animal. Older members might be given the opportunity to project themselves into a story of

"What if…" or "In ten years' time, I'll live in another country/on another planet where things are different."

5.    The group leader can tell a story and then invite group members to deconstruct it. Who were the important people in the story? Why? What role did they play that impacted on the story line? How would the story have changed if they had been different? Shuffle different characters of the story into different roles. Elaborate on how they may have acted differently and why (make connections between motivations and behaviors, looking at different perspectives). How can we tell what sort of characters they have? We haven't seen them, just heard words about them. What words can be used to suggest that this is someone you would like or not like?

## 5.15 Let me tell you about the movie I saw

Oral story.

### Objective

To tell a story to a conversation partner.

### Implementation

1.    Group members form pairs.

2.    Each tells a story that has a timeline, according to sequence, in a cohesive manner, relating links to each other, discarding extraneous information.

3.    Conversation partner can politely indicate when he or she is geting bored or lost, and practice listening skills by retelling the story. What was the essence, the main storyline?

Variations on this activity which practices speaking and listening skills, depending on level, are:

-    My first memory.

-    An experience that changed my life.

-    Someone who has inspired me (discussion of "inspiration" – how it could relate to gratitude, one of the strengths for resilience).

## 5.16 Stories of perspective

Storytelling, puppets, drama.

### Objective

Understand different perspectives of the same situation.

### Implementation

1.  Identify a situation where a number of people (parallel to the number of members in the group) have different perspectives. For example, there may have been an accident. Representing an unbiased perspective, a policeman controls the drama of different perspectives by asking each person in turn what they saw, heard, believed about the accident. One group member might have driven the car that hit the bike, another may have been a boy on the opposite side of the road playing with his friends, another will be the person whose leg is broken and is lying patiently waiting to be treated. The goal of this part of the exercise is to:

    *   identify that other perspectives are different but valid.

    *   realise that sometimes a clear picture only emerges when all perspectives are taken into consideration – one perspective is often misleading and not enough to establish "the truth."

2.  In social situations, an AS individual can be very dominating. He or she can act like the star of the show. Interruptions and insensitivity to the needs of others can be the result. Perspective stories can be used to illustrate that life is a show where everybody is the star to some extent and that we are all sharing the stage. Illustrate this with a simple drama requiring a number of people on a crowded stage and one actor taking up so much physical space that he pushes someone else off into the "orchestra pit." It might be illustrated with a choir where one person sings louder than all of the others; playing music where one instrument dominates and drowns out the others. Parents may offer examples of when an individual constantly interrupts or dominates family life. Stories can be individualized to specific situations and the perspectives of specific people. "What did Mom see, hear, and feel?" "What did Dad see, hear, and feel?"

    If drama is being employed in groups, analogies can be drawn: "On the kitchen stage at home, did one person crowd out the other players, not listen to them, respect their point of view, or try to understand their experience?" "We all crowd out others sometimes, without meaning to. What are examples – looking back – when you may not have listened to other people well, or understood their experience?"

3.  Use these principles in an art-related activity. If everybody is sharing one piece of paper and each is contributing to the same image, what happens if someone (predetermined) takes a heavy black pen and makes marks into everybody else's space? How does that make the other artists feel?

## 5.17 Story sequencing

Cartoon story.

### Objective

Understand the essence of a story, be able to reorganize it without losing sequence or meaning. Cooperation and teamwork.

### Implementation

A story or cartoon is read. Cut up a printed copy of the story or cartoon into ten, twelve, or appropriate number of pieces.

1.  Work together to reassemble it in the right sequence.
2.  If the story is broken into three parts, where would the breaks be made?
3.  If there is a moral to the story, what is it?
4.  Retell the story, cutting out 50 percent of the sentences and keeping the essence as much as possible.
5.  If the story was to be told in pictures, what would be the most important visual components of the story in any given place? (For example, when Goldilocks is found in bed by the three bears, what are the most important components? The quilt on the bed or facial expressions?)

## 5.18 Imaginative stories

Story, art.

### Objective

Make up surreal stories that stretch the imagination, maintaining sequence and a cohesive storyline.

## Implementation

ACTIVITY #1

1.  Start with:

    - Mr. Mrs. Miss…
    - Went to…
    - And…
    - She saw…
    - And decided to…
    - Then Mr. Mrs. Miss… came along
    - And said…, etc.

2.  Step 1 can be modified by telling a story in a round. Each person adds something to the story and passes a token object to the next person when they have finished and it is their neighbor's turn. The goal is to be imaginative, move the story but within a cohesive whole. There must be a sense of beginning, movement, conclusion with common threads, some repetition, some "point."

ACTIVITY #2

1.  Remove approximately five pictures from a container (with eyes closed).

2.  Use the pictures as elements of a cohesive story.

## 5.19 Moral stories

Stories, drama.

## Objective

Identify concept, implications.

## Implementation

1.  Some stories have a "moral." Read one similar to that below. (Using an interesting or surreal visual image or visually funny story supports memory.)

    *Valuing differences and working together*
    Two young men wanted to travel to Africa to see the lions. Unfortunately one was blind and the other had no legs. But when they met each other they became friends and decided to go to Africa together. Other people thought they looked a bit funny – the blind man carrying his friend and the man without legs giving his friend directions. But it worked for them.

One day, on a safari, the group they were traveling with was attacked by a rogue elephant. The man with no legs, who was sitting on the shoulders of the blind man at the time, yelled, "Run! Run!" Unfortunately, in his excitement he forgot to give directions. When the elephant saw this strange creature, nine foot high with two heads, fearlessly rushing toward it and yelling "Run! Run!" it got such a fright, it turned around and ran back into the jungle. Everyone was saved and the two friends were heroes. Together, they had power that others can only dream about.

## ACTIVITY #1
Discussion:

- What is the moral of the story?
- How can the moral be generalized (applied) to different and real-life situations?
- Do you sometimes feel different to other people? How?
- What are some of the good things about parts of yourself that are different to other people?
- Everybody is different in their own way. What is unusual about your friends and what do you like about those things?

## ACTIVITY #2
Ask group members to tell a story with a "message" or a "moral." Perhaps family members can help them find a story and relate the moral to the group. Help group members make up their own story with a "message" or "moral."

- What are some morals around which you could build a story? (Example: "It pays to be honest." "All that glitters is not gold.")
- Draw a story from your own experience.
- Make up a story.
- Finish it with the sentence: "And the moral of that story is…"

## ACTIVITY #3
From a list of morals or proverbs (example below), choose one to relate to real-life experiences. Write and enact a short drama that demonstrates and applies the moral of a story:

- The best things in life are free.
- United we stand, divided we fall.
- If a job's worth doing, it is worth doing well.
- Better to be alone than in bad company.
- Two wrongs don't make a right.

## 5.20 Combining talents

Story, paper activity.

### Objective

Value the uniqueness of self and others. Teamwork.

### Implementation

1.  Referring to the story in activity 5.17 about the two friends on safari, if you combined your unusual talents with the unusual talents of your friends, what could you do together? What interesting stories could you make up about that?

2.  Each person is given a different piece of paper on which to write. Write a list of the things you are interested in, your talents, or your skills. Include things you would like to be talented in or plan to be talented in one day.

3.  Cut your list up so that each interest, talent, or skill is on a separate piece. Put all the pieces of paper in the middle of the table – each person on a different piece of paper.

4.  Now pull out three pieces of paper of different colors – a piece of paper from each person. Using at least one word from each of the colors, have the group construct a story or an invention using a combination of the words pulled from the center of the table. Be as surreal as you dare. The only limit is your imagination.

# Symbols

Language is most expressive and more powerful when it uses metaphor, symbol, and analogy. Just as a picture is worth a thousand words, use of a symbol or metaphor offers a great deal of information. A symbol can also be used to represent a concept (green has political implications for some people; see also "Different caps: different perspectives," earlier in this chapter.

An important part of supporting AS is to provide non-conventional, non-concrete, and expansive tools for processing and expression. Even when it is difficult for individuals with AS to adopt a symbolic, non-literal way of thinking, it is important to understand the role analogies can play in other people's conversation.

## 5.21 Symbols: feelings and concepts

Art.

### Objective

To reflect on feelings, concepts, and represent them in symbolic terms. There are no wrong answers in this exercise. Validate everyone's opinion and input.

### Implementation

1.  Look at the introduction activity (4.1) which uses pictures to describe self, perhaps in symbolic ways. Using magazine pictures, painted pictures, found objects, practice using symbolism. If I said I was like a rock, what might that mean? If I painted myself with lots of sharp lines, like a porcupine, what might that mean? If I painted myself in a tiny square in the corner of a large piece of paper, what might that mean?

2.  Make a list of words or terms that could be used to describe what is important to you – thoughts, feelings, things.

3.  Represent those thoughts, feelings, and other things about you and in your life with symbols. For example, a feeling of sadness could be represented by a tear. The thought that "I am not liked" could be represented by a single flower alone and lonely, or a single black square (mood color). The thought that "I am popular" could be represented by a group of yellow flowers with one blue one in the middle. Discussion: What would represent a family to you? Or happiness? Or a good future?

4.  Draw or paint the symbols, transfer to clay tiles or paper.

## 5.22 Symbols in rituals

Discussion.

### Objective

Use symbols and rituals for emotional expression.

### Implementation

Individuals with Asperger's Syndrome typically enjoy rituals. They are familiar, repetitive, predictable, reassuring. Typically, they are not as comfortable with symbols or expression of emotions. Integrating symbols with rituals opens up potential for therapeutic strategies. Existing rituals can be modified (bedtime stories can be personalized to give opportunities to express personal feelings and experiences; early morning time normally spent on one's own can be used to write a journal); or new rituals can be constructed (a card is given to each group member to celebrate a success in one of their goals; a squeeze ball can be used to "get the anger out").

1. Let's look at rituals. Rituals are patterns of behavior. What are seasonal rituals in your home? Are they similar or different to the rituals in other homes? What about birthdays, Sunday mornings, holidays? What other rituals or patterns of behavior are there in your house?

2. What personal rituals or habits do you have? What do you like about them?

3. The group facilitator asks:

   - If I wave my country's flag, am I showing support for my country or a lack of respect for it?

   - I was born in Australia but live in America. Why is a koala bear hanging from the mirror in my car?

   - Why do some people wear their team's favorite colors?

   - If I give my friend Sandy a flower, am I offering her peace or showing my anger?

   - My sister turned 21 recently and my father gave her a key but it doesn't fit any door. Why did he give her the key?

   - Why did her boyfriend give her a friendship ring?

   - My mother keeps a scrapbook with photos of important days in our lives. Why does she do that?

   - When we visit Grandma, we have "tea," even though we don't really like tea. Why does she do that?

   In all of these things, objects are used to demonstrate our feelings about something. I miss Australia but I can't carry it around with me, photographs bring back lots of good feelings for past times for Mom, and it is hard to offer peace except with a symbol. Grandma uses tea as a ritual for the family to sit down together and talk to each other. The tea itself isn't important, it is a symbolic ritual. Can you think of examples where people use symbols or symbolic rituals in their lives?

4. Sometimes we use symbols to say something when words aren't enough. We use symbols to represent something too big to carry around (like Australia) or something that is just an idea, not real (like "freedom" or "friendship"). Symbols can also be very useful to put feelings into. It is better to kick a wall than kick a friend when we're angry. Sometimes it is useful to express feelings through symbols. We can put our worry into worry beads, put our anger into a rock and throw it into a river, put good wishes into a present and give it to a friend. Some people have put

their feelings into letters and then burned the letters rather than sending them to real people. They've been able to express their feelings even when and if the other person didn't hear about them.

Think of some examples of feelings that cause trouble – they are too big to handle or sometimes you just don't know what to do with them. Here are some examples:

- Your best friend is going to go to another school. What symbol could you give to him to carry in his pencil case so he remembers you at the new school?

- You really enjoy a particular band. What symbol could you carry with you to remind you of the band and show people how much you like them?

- You get really angry sometimes. How could you use a symbol to manage your own anger?

- Life gets tough sometimes but you hope that it will be better in the future. What symbol could you use and carry with you to represent a better future and to give you hope?

5. How can symbols be used in the group?

  - How could you use a symbol in a welcoming ritual? (A ritual is a pattern of behavior.)

  - How could you use a symbol to give people in the group permission to talk?

  - How could you use a symbol to show people they are going off track in conversation? (You might be using one already – forming a T with your hands.)

6. Designing your own symbols and rituals. Sometimes as we move through life we move through invisible milestones. In times past, maturity was celebrated for a young African man when he first killed a lion. Now stages are celebrated with graduation ceremonies and birthday parties. Sometimes, however, we pass stages in our lives that are important to us but nobody else knows about them or makes a fuss. They might include reaching personal secret goals, saving a particular amount of money, reaching a particular level of expertise in music or debating, completing a project or collection.

   What are some things in your life that you would like to achieve? What are achievements in your life that you would like other people to know about or celebrate? How can these achievements be marked? How can you celebrate achieving different stages or levels? (Finishing small steps and stages can be just as important as completing a goal and celebrating them might help you through the longer process. Symbolic rituals can provide the punctuation points for our lives.)

Sometimes we have difficulties in expressing ourselves. I knew a very intelligent man who stuttered. But when he used puppets to express what he felt, he didn't stutter at all. Sometimes, holding something, or putting our feelings through something else, helps us get them out more easily. It is almost as if those symbolic things give us permission to do what we have difficulty doing on our own.

Do you have difficulty talking about something? Try talking through something – through a puppet or behind a mask. Do you have difficulty showing your anger, courage, disappointment, fear, love? Would it help to express them to something else or in another place? Sometimes groups provide "a safe place" to express feelings. What other "safe places" are there in your life?

Sometimes we have feelings that we can't express because it is impossible to deal directly with the person involved (I am sad that my grandmother has died and I can't tell her how much I miss her) or it is inappropriate (I hate my teacher but can't tell him that). Sometimes we have bad feelings inside us and there is no one to direct them at (anger, pain, emptiness, guilt, feelings about the past). When we can't get hurtful feelings out of our bodies, they can make us sick. Sometimes those feelings get transferred into other behaviors that are not helpful to you (crying about Grandma, talking back in class because you don't like the teacher).

Do you have unfinished business with someone? Do you have feelings and it is impossible to express them to the person you have feelings about? Can you transfer those feelings into a symbolic object to get them out of your body where they can be hurtful and destructive?

Janine Roberts (1999) suggests that we don't have to design new rituals for ourselves. We can use existing ones. If we used to walk on the beach with Grandma and she has passed on, we might find ways to express our feelings about her during walks on the beach now.

Sometimes, without thinking about it, we adopt other people's rituals and they are not helpful to us. Many adolescents think they have to drink or take drugs to "have a good time." Often, though, it is because they haven't been creative or original enough to come up with different rituals for having a good time. (Some adolescents are so happy and tired from rock climbing or skin diving during the day, drinking at a party does not look like a good time.)

Sometimes there are cultural, family, and school rituals, habits, or "traditions" that we follow without thinking. Some rituals are good and uplifting, some bring us down. Identify some rituals that are not helpful to you or bring you down. Can you be creative and replace them with rituals or regular activities of your own?

Optimal conditions to encourage enjoyment of productive activities, autonomy, and individuality include challenging opportunities for individual expression in a context of warmth and support (Rathunde 2001).

## Symbolism and abstraction in art

Imagination is a strength for resilience and a difficulty for AS. AS artists often render wonderful realistic images but it is in effect copying, not drawing with a great deal of feeling.

## 5.23 Imaginative art

Mixed media.

### Objective

Build courage in communicating imaginative ideas.

Here are some strategies for art-related activities to build courage in communicating an imaginative idea, not realistic, abstract, to be interpreted.

### Implementation

Try new, novel materials and combinations:

- finger painting on found objects
- use the non-dominant hand
- making art with feet (use bare feet in different materials – also good for sensory integration) or other parts of the body
- stamp with found objects, identifying a shape in nature (fat triangles in hills, skinny triangles in trees, interlocking rectangles in buildings) and play with the shapes, turning them in different directions, laying them on top of each other.

# Motivation

> **Perseverance/industry/diligence**
> Three of the strengths that enhance resilience are perseverance, industry, and diligence. They are all grounded in motivation. What underlies motivation?

## 5.24 Motivation strategies

Cognitive restructuring, mind map.

### Objective

Clarify underlying factors in motivation.

### Implementation

The following are four reasons why motivation may be weakened and four strategies for bolstering motivation to get the job done. Read these strategies. Before you begin, you might identify a project that you must complete but have little enthusiasm for. As you read, apply the strategies to your example. Then invite group members to hypothetically use the strategies in real-life situations.

STRATEGY #1

Think of a project you are involved in or should be involved in but doesn't hold any interest for you. On a piece of paper write the name of the project and from that extend a line in one direction as one line in a spider mind. Along this line and at the end of it, illustrate the associations and feelings you have about it.

For our example, we will imagine it is a homework project that's going to take four weeks. This means you'll miss going to the shore with friends, movies, and generally hanging out. It means you'll have to get your act together, get down to the library, late nights, tired, miserable, resentful.

Emotions and goals work together to harness motivation (energy) and direction. If those emotions you have just illustrated are weakening your motivation, it makes sense that to get the job done you'll have to change your attitude. Oops, I mean you'll have to change your emotions.

Take a colored pen back to the center of your spider mind. The assignment is on history of music. Continue to think about your thoughts, feelings, and their associations. You like music, hate history – do a line to one edge of the paper – history, black hole, past, shredded paper, yuk, yuk, yuk. Spread black ink on it for good measure. So much for history.

Back to the center of your spider mind. What else do you associate with music history? Well, there's the music. That could lead to a line of lots of colors, notes, concerts, dinner last week with Susan before you went to a concert – she plays the violin, draw a violin – she's great – draw a smile – lots of happy colors here.

Back to the center of the spider mind. Still thinking about Susan's smile though…next line … This project is important. It is part of a final presentation. I wonder if Susan will come to see the final presentation. The history project could really tie it altogether. That's a good idea for the assignment. It could be related to the theme of the final presentation. Yes, I could relate it to the essay I did last September and the project I want to do next year. I can use it to tie the other assignments together.

And with newfound emotion (enthusiasm), motivation is born. Build a map of feelings, ideas, and associations. Connections, links, applications, and supportive ideas will be made. Inspiration (motivation) to continue the flow of creative ideas will come.

## STRATEGY #2

Motivation is likely to be weaker if involvement in a task is the result of external requirements and expectations. If a student is completing a project for course requirements and is not personally engaged, tenacity is likely to be less than if he or she makes a conscious connection with an end result (to finish the course by August, get a job, and make some money) or if there is a genuine interest (learn more about photography to take better photographs) and internal motivation (taking karate lessons to defend self).

Thoughts and beliefs about the reasons for doing a task are central to this aspect of motivation. One solution to the motivation challenge is to reorganize thoughts about a task and "take ownership" of it. Find a way to become personally engaged, to invest self, to gain something of personal value from it, or to connect it somehow to an area of genuine interest.

An application of this idea is to use the brainstorm/mind map format again to explore the theme of "personal satisfaction" or "personal reward." What is rewarding for each individual? Go beyond the immediate and obvious (money, games) to underlying factors (spending time with friends), associations (freedom, prestige), and what the individual would like more of (knowledge about something, working in partnership with other people). Discuss in the group how information from this exercise can be integrated with the project to create more enthusiasm.

## STRATEGY #3

The ability and skills to finish a task are important. Perhaps the individual really does not have the necessary skills but that is probably a rare situation. It is always possible to learn new skills, ask for help. It is more likely that a history of failures (no matter how seemingly insignificant) has left a person feeling pessimistic. They are not confident or capable and failure is a probability; or that any success is due to the teacher/parent/support, not their own effort. Again, motivation is a product of thoughts or beliefs more than expertise.

Self-awareness of strengths and confidence built from previous experiences will buffer a person in challenging tasks. Confidence and esteem grow to build self-efficacy, which in turn will directly affect motivation and related emotions, choices, and performance. A support system can significantly modify perceptions of efficacy with encouragement, feedback, and challenge of faulty beliefs.

Use group discussion to share ideas about who and what comprises a support system. Use the group to practice the social skill of interacting with others in a reciprocal and supportive manner, listening and building on integrated ideas. In pragmatic terms, what is needed for the individual to feel ready or skilled in something? How realistic is that? How close to reality are they now? What steps can be made to build the necessary skills and confidence to complete the project?

### STRATEGY #4

Finally, and most importantly for individuals with Asperger's Syndrome, motivation can be weakened considerably by an inability to plan, sequence, initiate appropriate techniques and strategies, and generally organize the task. Loss of motivation will be increased if the individual sees this as a personal character weakness – that he or she is at fault ("stupid") rather than that the task is too difficult.

It may be necessary to learn self-organization skills – timelines, organizational charts, and so on. These are tools that can be learned – not a reflection of someone's intelligence or character. Remember, three of the strengths that enhance resilience are perseverance, industry, and diligence. Use every opportunity to commend these qualities as personal strengths that are admirable and valuable. They provide the foundation for achieving goals.

### WHAT STRATEGY TO USE?

*What is a task you currently have difficulty being motivated with?* With any issue, supportive intervention must be tailored to individual needs and be situation specific. Make questions concrete and logical. Have them build on each other so that through answering the questions, the individual becomes more aware of underlying factors and is able to arrive at their own realistic conclusion. Questions might include:

- Why are you engaged in this task?
- For whom are you doing the task?
- What advantages are there in completing it? What will you get out of it?
- Do you feel you can complete the task?
- If not, why not? What evidence is there for that?

- What has motivated you to complete tasks in the past? What has caused you to give up?
- Do you have the necessary skills? What skills need to be learned?
- Can you use help in planning the necessary steps?
- Does it matter to you what other people think of you? Do you care if other people see you fail? (If making a good impression on others is important, an individual may not become involved in a challenging task in case of being seen to fail. The reluctance to accept the challenge might be manifested in other evasive or disruptive behavior. This is an opportunity to elaborate on the valuable personal skills of perseverance, industry, and diligence.)
- Do you see this task as making you a stronger, more knowledgeable person or just getting the job done? (Love of learning, another personal strength, and enjoyment of the task for itself, offer more resilience than performance-oriented behavior – also called intrinsic motivation.)

CHAPTER 6

# Self-awareness and self-related skills

## Emotion, depression, anxiety, emotional self-regulation

## Self-awareness

> Perhaps the single most useful objective in supporting an adolescent with Asperger's Syndrome is to increase self-awareness.

### 6.1 Initials

Expressive art, collage, etc.

*Objective*

Expression of individuality.

*Implementation*

Initials are familiar, unique, and personal. Making art with them allows a focus on the "how" rather than the "what."

Write your own initials, once or many times, in a way or ways that show yourself, your personality, the things you like and don't like – whatever you think is important about you and as much a part of you as your initials.

## 6.2 Personal story #1: life map

Expressive art, drawing, collage, etc.

### Objective

Graphically represent the "ups" and "downs" of life – an overview of perception of own life.

### Implementation

Using a drawing, a graph, timeline, or abstract map, draw the "ups" and "downs" of life up to this age. Represent different meaningful events along the way with pictures, symbols, or words.

## 6.3 Personal story #2: past, present, and future

Expressive art, collage.

### Objective

Introduce, build empathy within a group, clarify important elements about self, make connections between past, present, and future. This is a fundamental and important exercise. Each piece – past, present, and future – deserves at least a separate day for processing and expression.

### Implementation

1. Using paint, collage, expressive media of some kind, tell your personal story in three separate pieces of work.

2. The first piece tells the story of your past – early memories, surroundings, what and who was important to you. If you don't like to share everything with the group, include symbols that only you understand the meaning of. Use materials that have a layering effect (netting, pockets, envelopes) to represent some things hidden or nearly forgotten. You may use something that gives an impression of moving through time, from one place to another, or a change happening for you. Use materials that feel "right" and describe through touch and/or color the feelings associated with what you are describing. Feelings are an important part of the process.

3. The second part of this exercise (probably on another day) is to create another painting or collage that describes where you are now. Using imagination and materials in a creative, symbolic way, describe feelings

and relationships, cause and effect associations, and so on. Express what is important to you personally, even if you don't want to talk about it.

4.    The last part of this exercise is the future – not necessarily as you expect it to be but as you would like it to be. Again, focus on feelings, colors, textures to suggest something that you may not have easy words for.

5.    At each stage of this exercise, or after it has all been finished, discuss what you choose with other people. There is no need to share everything – everyone has the right to talk only about the things with which they are comfortable. If something arises in this exercise that makes you upset or uncomfortable, talk to the group leader in private about it.

6.    This activity can be extended by "wrapping" the pieces and using them in a book or personal story board; or applying to another two- or three-dimensional item.

## Photography

Technology offers wonderful opportunities to personalize art through photography in ways not available until recent years. Photo transfer paper allows photographs to be transferred from computer to fabric, wood, metal – the combinations are limitless. This is a particularly useful craft for individual support or very small groups with access to a reliable computer and digital photographic equipment. If using a computer is not convenient, use a mobile photo printer for digital cameras. Photographs of individuals with or without their friends can immediately be printed and included in creative activities.

Photo therapy is becoming a creative therapy in its own right. As activity 4.1 (Introductions) demonstrated, photography offers an opportunity for projection. The individual can project ideas that are important to him or her onto a photograph taken by somebody else, or choose to take a photograph of something that has unique meaning for him or her. Photographs may make direct reference to particular people and things and can also be used symbolically. They can offer unlimited and relevant information and still be aesthetically pleasing. They can be casual and spontaneous or formal and posed, representing the past or the present. The way a collage is put together and what it is used for can be as interesting as the information within any one photograph. Combined with other media, the potential of photography as a therapeutic technique has no boundaries.

For the individual with Asperger's Syndrome, integrating the view of self with the rest of the world, using photographs as a learning and support tool is logical and attractive. Having a digital camera and printer is invaluable in personalizing collages with personal stories.

## 6.4 Personal story #3: an event

Cartoon, script, puppets.

### Objective

To tell personal stories from an observer's perspective through use of puppets.

### Implementation

1. Choose something from your life that was funny, sad, or important to you. If you tell this story to someone else, identify what the essential message is that you want to get across. What are your feelings about this event? Do you want to share your feelings about it? Do you want your audience to feel a little bit what you were feeling or are feeling about it now?

2. Through cartooning or scriptwriting, make a story about it – beginning, introducing the people, place, situation; choosing elements that clearly signpost progress through the story (actions, movement, outcomes, significant conversations); identify the essence of the story (moral, outcome, revealing or pivotal conversations/actions) and don't go off at tangents. Keep to a sequence that has an appropriate beginning and end and moves smoothly between them.

3. Rehearse the story with puppets. Can you cut out unimportant details? Can you put more emphasis (movement, gesture, tone of voice) on a pivotal sentence or piece of action? Does the language you are using get the feelings you have about the story across to the listener? Can you use backdrop, props, music to add to the feelings of your story (humor, sadness and so on)? Sometimes they will be more effective than words alone. Don't rush – sometimes well-timed silences can be more effective than words. Give your audience time to think about the story as it happens.

4. After rehearsal, tell your story with puppets. Involve your audience by asking them for feedback. Did they understand the feelings you wanted to get across? What did they think were the most important elements? What impression did the props and non-verbal elements give? What did they learn about you? What can you learn from their feedback?

## 6.5 Self-awareness themes

Art, mind maps, fabric collage.

### Objective

Explore individuality.

### Implementation

1. Close your eyes and think about the following questions as they are read (questions should be read with time between them for reflection):

   - What does it feel like to be you?
   - What are the characteristics that describe you best?
   - How do you feel different to others?
   - What are the good things about your individuality/uniqueness?
   - What are the challenges about your individuality/uniqueness?
   - What are the colors and shapes and textures of feeling different?

2. Describe your feelings about your individuality through expressive art (collage, paint, sculpture).

3. Do a spider map with "individuality" being the central theme. Write and draw whatever comes to mind. Where can your individuality take you?

4. Other group members write three things that are individual and positive that they appreciate about you. Pin on shirt or develop into a keepsake "book."

5. Everybody's hands are unique. Some say that hands indicate character and even the direction our lives will take. Using your hand as a template, develop a piece of art that expresses the uniqueness of you.

6. Add to the hand in ways that describe your individuality and uniqueness.

   - Make a collage with hands from the group.
   - As a variation of the theme, use fabric (backed with iron-on adhesive) and fabric pens and paints and make a fabric collage. The finished piece of fabric could be used to make an individualized tote bag or similar (see Figure 8.5).

7. Another variation of this theme is to explore individuality of self through photographs. Use old photos, take new photos. Choose colors and symbols and photographs that represent parts of you that are important to you, and other people, pets, interests, and things in your world that contribute to your individuality and uniqueness.

## 6.6 Themes relating to self and emotions

Expressive art, collage, fabric collage, and/or mind maps.

### Objectives

Exploring failures; laziness, apathy, boredom; energy.

### Implementation

**FAILURES**

Use a mind map to explore the emotions around failures. Use images, colors, and lines to express what failure feels like. When you've failed, how important was it to you? Why? How can failures have an ongoing impact? There is a saying "In every cloud there is a silver lining." What does that mean and was there a silver lining in your failure?

**LAZINESS, APATHY, BOREDOM**

Is there a connection between physical and emotional feelings? For example, do you suddenly feel very tired when you have to clean your room? How can you use this information to get more energy?

Use a spider map to explore the things that drain you of energy, that make you feel lazy or bored. What emotions do you share with those things? How can you turn this knowledge into a positive tool for yourself?

**ENERGY**

This is the mirror activity for the one on laziness, apathy, boredom.

Using a spider map, is there a connection between physical and emotional feelings? For example, do you suddenly feel energized when a friend calls and suggests going to the movies (or a place that you enjoy)? What emotions are associated with energy? Anticipation? How can you use this information to put more energy into things that otherwise would be a drain for you? Explore possibilities with a spider map. (Be silly, funny, inventive, imaginative.)

### Self-awareness themes

All activities don't have to be formally structured. Sometimes a "casual" conversation during snack time can lead to meaningful food for thought. The following themes and questions can be modified to suit skill level and available time. They might be themes for discussion (spontaneous or "passing the baton") or they may provide subject matter for art, scriptwriting, improvised skits, mind maps, and so on.

- Emptiness
- Gratefulness
- Dreams
- Sadness, happiness
- Embarrassment
- Fear, stress, anxiety
- Loss
- Loss and growth
- Growth
- Self-discipline, regulation
- Success
- Integrity
- Moodiness
- Feeling different
- Loneliness
- Procrastination
- Strengths and weaknesses
- Flexibility, inflexibility
- Self-centeredness
- Positive behavior, destructive behavior
- Self-development, personal goals
- What's the best thing that's happened to you?
- What are you looking forward to most?
- What worries you most?
- What really annoys you most? What makes you most angry? And what's the difference between being annoyed and being angry for you?
- Five of the best things about you
- Five of the worst things about you

- How have you changed in the last two years/since going to that school/since coming to this group?
- Why do you think you've changed?
- Do you expect to keep changing through your life?
- What are some changes you'd like to make or see?
- When it's a good idea to keep secrets
- The best thing (or things) about AS
- The worst thing (or things) about AS
- What makes you happiest?
- Things would be better in your life if...

## Interests

**Zest/passion/enthusiasm – hope/optimism/future-mindedness**
These qualities have been identified as being personal strengths that enhance resilience. Great opportunity for those with Asperger's Syndrome! Temple Grandin stresses the importance of taking personal interests as a starting point for developing a career. Interests and obsessions signpost a future about which an individual can be optimistic, enthusiastic, and even passionate.

## 6.7 Personal interests/career potential

Mind maps, Three-Step Plan.

### Objective

Explore personal interests and potential associations with future using alternative ways of processing – spider maps, thinking hats, Three-Step Plan.

### Implementation

1. Using the Three-Step Plan (5.4) and one or a combination of the above creative techniques, explore interests and associations.
2. Collect facts (including what you are interested in, what skills you have, how old you are, how many years you have to execute your plan for a future career, current and projected market demand for your skills);

reasons and motivation for developing personal interests and possible career now.

3.    Explore possibilities, alternatives, options. Use creative and associative thinking. What are possible ways to develop personal interests (whether or not they may develop into a career), explore advantages, possible problems, creative solutions, look at it from the perspective of "If I didn't have to earn money" and "If I wanted to invent a completely new professional field"? Can you visit a professional or someone working in the area of your interest? Ask to interview them to see what their job is really like, what they do, what they like, what they don't like. What are the required personal skills and characteristics? Remember, in this step, the sky is the limit. Pay attention to your feelings and instincts.

4.    Given the information obtained from the previous step, what are the best decisions and choices? Convert this information back into a timeline and concrete steps, prioritized and sequenced. What are the short-term goals? What are the long-term goals? When looking at the concrete plan, what possible weak links are there? What preparations can be made to strengthen the weak links or prevent problems?

## 6.8 Developing personal interests/future possibilities

Discussion, art.

Discussion can take five minutes or be developed into expressive art activities.

### Objective

Expand and develop interests.

### Implementation

- What are three interests or skills you'd like to have or develop?
- What has stopped you from developing those interests?
- What practical, concrete steps can you take to develop those interests?
- What goal can you set for yourself in the next seven days to develop an interest? Report back to the group and support each other in ongoing development of goals.

## 6.9 Personal shield

Art, collage, sculpture, metalwork, printmaking.

Provide cardstock templates of possible shapes and layouts for a personal shield. Include space for words or a personal creed.

### Objective

Design and make a personal shield.

### Implementation

1. Imagine you have your own personal shield – like a knight in the medieval ages. Your shield has three or four images representing the things that are important to you, that describe you, or you would like to have one day (even if you don't like them now).

2. At the same time, imagine what your creed or personal mission statement might be. This shield represents the ideal you, the aspects of you (which may not be fully developed yet) that will give you strength and direction in your life. One or more of the images on the shield should relate to what you want to be (your character) and one or more of the images or creed should relate to what you want to do in your life.

3. Choose a craft that gives you pleasure to work with and will produce a long-lasting shield. It might be two-dimensional (paper and paint collage on cardstock) or three-dimensional (hammered metal, painted air dry clay).

4. Trace the outline of a shield onto your chosen material from a template. (Wrap metal edges with tape available from stained glass supply stores.) Divide the shield into three or four sections for the images, allow space for the creed.

5. Attach a hook behind or on top of the shield for hanging, or attach it to a base for standing.

6. Finish the shield with a glaze.

## 6.10 Personalized print

Printmaking.

A variation on the personal shield is the personalized stamp and print, similar to a monogram. Sometimes an exercise that allows expression of individuality, when repeated after a period of time, will demonstrate a change in self-perception.

*Objective*

Personalize a stamp.

*Implementation*

1.  Choose a medium suitable to the skill level of the group/individual. Linoleum or rubber tiles can be carved with tools available in craft shops. For those with less agile fine motor skills, use a wooden base and glue detail onto it (string, cut paper, textured materials – surface must be level to pick up ink).

2.  Remember that carving out a design will leave a negative space and a mirror image when printed.

3.  A simpler version of the monogram stamp is to let group members doodle their initials in variations for a much longer time than they would normally give it (20 or more minutes). Encourage use of new medium, different colors, attaching symbols and frames. Given time and permission to elaborate, most will extend the initials with which they are very familiar, through old boundaries to new places. At the same time, while hands are busy, faces down, and eyes averted, and concentration is not needed, the conversation is likely to wander away from the familiar task in hand and present new and interesting topics.

## 6.11 Self-portrait

All art.

*Objective*

Express perception of self-related themes in non-conventional ways.

*Implementation*

Through some form of expressive art – using any or all medium – do a self-portrait. It may be abstract or realistic. It is an exercise that can be repeated many times and is the starting point for discussion of different self-related themes.

This week, in a depressed mood, a self-portrait is likely to be much different to last week's portrait in a happy mood. Keeping a series of self-portraits is valuable for identifying growth and/or patterns.

# Masks

Masks have many of the same qualities as puppets. Designing them, making them, using them for a performance, all introduce a range of learning possibilities. In addition, masks are a more personal and direct way of self-expression. They provide the means for an individual to "act out" directly with freedom and creativity. Feelings are revealed and expressed while the actor feels protected and less vulnerable. Masks allow the integration of the person and a role they assume or is a less public aspect of themselves.

## 6.12 Mask of self

Collage, metal, other.

### Objective

To express individuality.

### Implementation

1. We all have many aspects of ourselves. Make a mask that illustrates what you look like on the outside. It might use symbols or colors or a design that communicates the way you want people to see you, or the way you think they do see you. Perhaps you wear different masks at home and school, with friends and people you don't know. With whom and under what conditions would you remove your mask?

2. Decorate the inside of the mask to reflect the inner, more private parts of yourself. You don't have to show the inside of the mask to anyone. Is the inside of the mask very different to the outside? If so, why do you think that is?

3. Ideas for making masks:

   - Foil covered with paper. Foil is molded around face, covered and strengthened with layers of paper and/or fabric.

   - Oven baked clay, available at craft stores.

   There are many ways and books on the subject of making masks. Cheap plastic masks, available at chain stores and party supply shops, are excellent value and convenient as a base to cover or decorate with paper, clay, fabric, or found objects.

> **Playfulness and humor**
> Playfulness and humor are strengths that enhance resilience.

## 6.13 If I was a bug

Three-dimensional craft.

### Objective

To have fun, use imagination, play.

### Implementation

1. If you were a bug, what would you look like? This activity is purely to laugh and have fun. It is an opportunity for you to design a surreal and way cool bug – and make up stories about it. "Its name is ... and he/she has ... because that reminds me of my..." and so on.

2. Make a body and head from air dried or oven baked clay, paper mâché, or scrunched up foil covered with paper.

3. Add legs and antennae out of wire twisted with pliers (twist around body); paint and decorate. Use beads for eyes, add swivels and wire, springs, beads, pieces of metal, fabric – whatever grabs the imagination.

4. Add wings if you like, by twisting wire in the shape of wings (allow extra length to twisted wire to attach to the body); wrap the wire wings with transparent or other paper; glue and glaze.

5. A variation on this is to portray other people as bugs. This activity gives the opportunity to express feelings in unconventional (often revealing) ways, while having fun.

## Mandalas

The mandala is a traditional form of art, often with spiritual and symbolic significance. It is usually in the form of a circle and represents the "self." Carl Jung believed the mandala could be used to express and explore "the wholeness of the personality" and enhance personal growth, realization, and transformation. Aesthetically, the mandala provides a stable, ordered, and pleasing structure which can be fragmented into "parts of the whole." Making a mandala is a form of active meditation.

Variations on this theme are endless. Mandalas may be tiny, on clay earrings or beads, or a larger size, perhaps a T-shirt or chalk on a cement floor. They can be pretty and symmetrical, or abstract and dramatic. They may be made with all the medium available, temporary traditional sand art mandalas, or permanent with clay, fabric, metal.

Because of the circle form that brings unity to smaller pieces, this is a pleasing design to apply to a quilt or wall hanging. The colors in fabric can also be used well in a mandala or kaleidoscope effect. There is a form of quilting piecing called "kaleidoscope" which would lend itself to this exercise for appropriate individuals.

Paint/draw a mandala on shrink plastic. Shrinking it with a heat gun will make it even more compact and graphic, suitable for jewelry, key rings, tiles, pieces for collage and decoupage.

## 6.14 Self-complexity mandala

All art.

One of the keys to resilience is complexity of self-concept – the number and range of roles that make up how a person sees themselves; and the interests and activities that take up their time, introducing new people, elements, and influences, and providing associated benefits. For people whose AS traits impact heavily on their lives, assistance in building a variety of activities and roles is very important.

The self-complexity mandala activity is designed to identify many aspects of the individual, acknowledge their importance, the contribution they make, and the influence they have.

### Objective

Identify self-aspects/identities/roles.

### Implementation

1.  With a basic circular template, such as a very large plate, draw a circle on paper. This will be the foundation for your mandala.

2.  Within the circle, make a random or symmetrical pattern, segmenting the circle, as simple or as complex as desired. Use the sections to contain different aspects of self, represented with lines, colors, textures, symbols, words – whatever is pleasing to you.

3.  "Aspects of self" might be external roles, such as mother, student, dog owner. They might be internal or dormant, such as lover of astronomy,

non-working artist. If they are an important part of you (even if they're dormant, sleeping), give them a place in the mandala. Some aspects may refer to emotions in your life – fearful, ambitious. Make associations with the roles and self-aspects. Not all sections have to be filled. Some sections may contain only color, some symbols, texture, print. There is no rule about staying within the lines and that means the boundary of the circle itself.

4. On completion, spend some time studying your mandala before discussing it with anyone else.

5. Questions: Are you surprised at the number of aspects of yourself? Is the mandala very busy? Are there many empty spaces? Were there many "sleeping" aspects of you? Are there aspects of yourself that go outside the boundary? What does that mean to you? Do you have control over most of your roles or are they determined by other people and circumstances (you have to go to school, you would prefer not to)? Are most of your roles satisfying? Do they have a positive influence on your life? Look at the balance of self-aspects. Is there a pattern? Does it lean heavily in one direction? For example, if playing sport is a large part of yourself what will happen when you leave school? Will you find other opportunities to find sport? Do many parts of yourself depend on being a student? What is left when you leave school?

6. The reasoning behind this activity is that people with a variety of self-aspects, interests, and identities have more to help them bounce back from difficult circumstances, when things and people in life change or fail or move on. Is there a part of you that is so important that if it was taken away or collapsed it would be extremely difficult for you? Looking at your mandala, is there anything you can do to strengthen interests and parts of yourself to make your life more balanced and resilient? What parts of you will help you when things go wrong, if life gets difficult? Even when circumstances knock you about, what parts of you will survive? Remember: Being authentic to ourselves is a core component to resilience. Topic for discussion during the activity may be the need to find a path between being ourselves and compromising for other people.

## 6.15 Self collage

Collage.

### Objective

Identify self aspects/identities/roles.

*Implementation*

Using the same questions as the mandala, do a free-form collage which puts the individual in the middle of the picture. Around the central image, identify aspects of self – "little selves," self at different ages, self in different places and roles, self from different perspectives.

## 6.16 Inner and outer me

Box, altered book.

*Objective*

Self-awareness; private and public aspects of self.

*Implementation*

1.  Make a three-dimensional collage out of a box or altered book (old book, cut hole/s out of pages which are then glued together, effectively forming a box between the book covers).

2.  On the outside of the box or book, use collage materials/paint etc. to describe the part of you which the rest of the world sees – the public face.

3.  On the inside of the box or book, use materials to describe the inner part of you which the world, or most of the world, does not see.

4.  There may be some definition between the boundaries with things hanging cut or the box/book partly open or a transparent window. There is potential for windows and many different sides.

## Strengths

Appendix 1 lists the names and descriptions of 24 strengths.

## 6.17 My strengths

Discussion and homework.

### Objective

Identify signature strengths.

### Implementation

1. Discuss the list of 24 strengths in Appendix I so that they are understood in terms appropriate to skill level. Simplify the list to key words and on another piece of paper write what you think are the five most applicable to you.

2. During the course of a week, give the list to a variety of people you know – parents, teachers, friends – and ask them to tell you which five they think are most pertinent to you.

3. At the end of the week, compare the response of different people with your own beliefs. Are they similar? What have you learned about yourself and the way other people see you?

4. How do you use your strengths? How could you use your strengths?

## 6.18 Self-discovery tour

Collage, self-expressive art.

### Objective

Identify strengths appreciated by self, strengths appreciated in other people, support network, goals.

### Implementation

1. Imagine you are setting out on a long journey. Your destination is important to you. It's something you want to see or do very much. Perhaps it's a goal for your future, something you'd like to know more about or experience. This won't be an easy journey – you can expect to meet a lot of new people, see new things, and be in dangerous and difficult situations. You will have to really want what's at the end of your journey to keep you going. What would you really like to experience, what would you like to learn or know more about, or do, one day?

2. Before you go, on a large piece of paper, draw or paint where you are now. Use symbols to describe where you are now.

3. As you go, you are told you can choose three personal strengths to help you through the difficult times. Which of your personal strengths or traits do you think would be most useful?

4.  Before you leave, you are also told you can choose a present for yourself to help you on your way. What do you think you would choose?

5.  If you could choose a traveling companion – someone you know or someone you don't know – who would it be? Why?

6.  Your first stop on the journey will be to collect knowledge that might help you. What knowledge do you need and who would be able to help you get that knowledge? Draw stop number one with symbols to represent the knowledge or things you need and the person or people who can help you get them on your journey.

7.  Your journey might require just one or two stops, it might require a number of stops, years, and a lot of effort. As much as possible, draw the journey, the stops, or steps you need to make to get to the destination. Some of the stops, or links in the chain of the journey, might include learning new skills to help you along the way, acquiring knowledge and tools, books on a particular subject, organizations that could help or that you could join.

8.  What will some of the obstacles be? How can your strengths help you? Write or draw the people who can help you as you go.

9.  What will the destination be like? What will be there? Who will be there? How will you feel? Draw a picture of the end of the journey.

10. When you've completed your journey, reorganize the information to make a poster that will be a visual reminder of where you want to go, and the strengths and steps that must be nurtured now to get to your goal. Appreciate the things and people around you that can help you get there.

## Emotions

Decoding emotions should play a part in every support activity. For the AS individual it is important to understand them, articulate them, and be able to modify them if necessary, rather than be controlled by them.

### *Journaling*

The purpose of a journal is to increase consciousness, a sense of continuity and pattern. It can be adapted for a variety of exercises (goal organization, relationship dynamics, satisfying activities). For the individual with AS traits, increasing consciousness of activities and thoughts offers a detached perspective, allows patterns to be identified and choices to be considered rather than being in "automatic mode." In discussion in groups, the differences and similarities in priorities, interests, and dislikes can add to group cohesiveness.

## 6.19 Making journals

Journal.

### Objective

Increase consciousness of activities and thoughts.

### Implementation

1.  Supply group members with easily carried notebooks (spiral notebooks are ideal). Make a project of individualizing their covers. If group members don't like writing, or don't have time, just a date, time, and a few key words will suffice. Use colored drawing materials if possible.

2.  Use the journal to document activities and how important they are for each individual. Why do we do the things we do? Why do we choose to spend our time as we do? Is it planned or do we just "go with the flow" and what feels good at the time? Do our activities contribute to long-term goals? Do we spend most of our time in activities of short-term pleasure? (We are not making moral judgments with this exercise – it is for the purpose of being conscious and aware of how we spend our time, and the repercussions of how we spend our time.)

    In Chapter 8 ("Nuts and bolts of art techniques"), ideas are suggested for constructing simple books or journals – also helpful in keeping together different activities, collages, writing, and art related to the same theme.

## 6.20 My emotions

Discussion.

### Objective

Identify emotions in our lives and their influence. The list can be modified as needed, appropriate to theme.

## Implementation

- Hope
- Sadness
- Happiness
- Excitement
- Disappointment
- Wonder
- Disgust
- Friendship

- Acceptance
- Fear
- Love
- Hate
- Amusement
- Kindness
- Courage
- Calmness

- Regret
- Guilt
- Shame
- Frustration
- Jealousy
- Envy
- Confidence
- Patience

Go through this list of emotions and write beside each one:

1. In what circumstances do you experience the emotion?
2. How often do you experience it?
3. How does each emotion influence other parts of your life?
4. Which are positive emotions and which are negative?
5. How are emotions helpful or unhelpful?
6. Do we control our emotions? Do our emotions control us?
7. People around you have some of these emotions too. When do they affect you?
8. How do your emotions affect other people?

## 6.21 Looking at emotions

Collage, expressive art.

### Objective

Identify emotions in our lives and their influence.

### Implementation

What do different emotions "look" like? Can you give them a shape or a color? Are they big in your life or little? What causes these emotions? Are there other emotions associated with those emotions? (This activity will help explore activity 6.20.)

## 6.22 Categorize emotions

Spider map, collage.

### Objective

To identify range of emotions, compare and contrast them. Categorize (conceptual thinking).

### Implementation

1. On a large piece of paper, write the names of different emotions – group them according to emotions that you think are similar, overlap, go together.

2. Explore each group with associations (when/where/how these are likely to be experienced).

3. Identify their common characteristics. Common source? Common outcome?

## 6.23 Explore being happy

Journal.

There is evidence that positive emotions and being happy provide a foundation for resilience. When we are happy we are more adaptable, open to learning, and resilient. There are different types of happiness and causes for happiness, some with more staying power than others.

This exercise builds tools for empowerment. It helps the individual understand how they can make positive and empowering choices for themselves, and the likely consequences of positive choices.

Because each step is important, they may be addressed at different times, and perhaps integrated into other activities. The principles are worth reiterating at different times and in different ways.

There is a heavy degree of discussion in this exercise but the Asperger individual typically likes to talk about self-related subjects. Telling stories about real-life examples can be an effective form of learning about the concept of happiness.

### Objective

Understand the power of happiness, be aware of the value of "gratification."

## Implementation

1. For a month, keep a journal that records the feelings and thoughts associated with different daily experiences. Record experiences of motivation and satisfaction. It is also helpful to identify areas associated with discomfort (such as socially demanding situations), areas of enjoyment (on the computer), or times when mood can be affected by physical factors (hunger or noise).

2. What makes you happy? Are you with particular people or doing particular things when you are at your happiest? If you were to choose three activities or things to make you happy, what would you choose? Is there anything new or different you'd like to do because you think it would make you happy?

3. Tell the group a story from your life about an occasion when you were unhappy. What stopped the unhappiness? When the unhappiness was removed, what did it feel like? Did you feel relieved? Did you feel happy? Did you feel nothing? Does removing something that makes you unhappy make you happy?

4. What do you need to be very happy? Close your eyes, imagine you have those things or are in that place. You have everything you need to make you happy. Imagine it for a minute. See it, feel it, hear it. What does it feel like? Discuss the feelings of happiness and identify differences between people. What makes other people happy and how does it feel for them?

5. What are the different types of happiness that you can feel? Compare visiting your grandmother with getting a high grade in your exam or being on a winning team. Do they feel different physically? Do some sources of happiness last longer than others? Does it make you happy to meet a challenge successfully? Make lists of the different things that make you happy and the different ways happiness can feel. On those lists, try to remember how long the different feelings of happiness last. If you cheer when your team wins, how long do you cheer for? How long would it be before your attention goes somewhere else? What if you missed your bus and had to walk home in the rain after the game? Does being happy mean always having a smile on your face? What is the difference between feeling happy and feeling good about something, about yourself?

6. Look at your lists. Do some types of happiness last longer than others? Which things make you happy but the feelings only last a short time? Which things make you happy but the feelings last a long time?

    Look at this list of pairs and discuss the different feelings that you think each activity would give you. How long do the feelings last?

Listening to a CD   •   Playing a guitar

Watching football on television   •   Football with friends

Playing a video game   •   Designing a video game

One of the differences in each pair is that one activity is "passive" and one requires participation, effort, challenge, learning, producing something, or long-term reward. Can you add to the list of pairs?

7.  Usually, things aren't all good or all bad. Most experiences can make us happy or sad, depending on what we focus on. (I had to stay home during summer but I learned to swim; my team always loses but it has great cheerleaders.) Sometimes the things that make us happy can help us deal with things that make us unhappy. Can you think of examples in your own life? Share them with the group.

8.  Now that you have gone through some or all of the listed items, the overall goal of the activity is to identify the deep-seated things that help you bounce back from unhappy experiences, the things that make you resilient in the face of unhappy things (item 7). Some books say that the types of happiness that come from good times, parties, watching a movie, and eating a good meal are nice but they don't last. These things are often connected to our senses (food–taste; hearing–music; sight–movies). They tend to melt away quickly – just like the sweets or candy we put in our mouths.

Longer lasting happiness (or satisfaction) comes from meeting challenges like learning something new or building a good friendship or designing a website. (Look again at the activities identified in item 6 that require participation and effort.) This type of activity is more likely to result in "flow." Flow is a feeling when you are so interested in what you are doing that you forget the time. You might feel a challenge but you also feel satisfaction because you are meeting the challenge.

This kind of happiness doesn't go away in a hurry. It can even help you when unhappy things happen. If you are having problems finding part-time work, eating sweets and watching movies won't help much. There will be more satisfaction in knowing that you're clever enough to build your own website (even if it doesn't get you the job delivering pizzas) and you have a friend you can share things with.

What do you think about this? Can you think of real-life examples when you experience flow? What kind of things in your life give you a resilient kind of happiness that helps you deal with unhappy things? Look at item 6. Which of these activities would have the power to help you feel better about yourself or to get through not-so-happy times?

9.  What things can you do in your life to make yourself happier? Which things will be fleeting and transient? Which things would have a long-term

effect and won't go away even when other things make you unhappy? What are some positive, challenging, and satisfying goals that you can set for yourself (short term and long term)? What personal strengths and interests do you have that you can develop to produce a sense of satisfaction, a deep-seated happiness that will not melt away easily? What goals can you set, activities can you do, skills can you develop that will empower you?

## 6.24 An open face

Role play.

### Objective

Show an "open face" with a range of emotions.

### Implementation

People tend to respond more positively to us if we show an "open face." Showing an open face means showing on our face what we are feeling inside.

In pairs, show your partner how you would show these emotions on your face. See how many they can guess.

| | | |
|---|---|---|
| • Sadness | • Hope | • Relief |
| • Happiness | • Kindness | • Regret |
| • Excitement | • Disgust | • Depression |
| • Disappointment | • Friendship | • Frustration |
| • Surprise | • Anger | • Fear |

If you have problems with this exercise – for example, showing sadness without contorting your face in an unnatural manner – practice it until it becomes more natural. It helps other people understand what you are feeling without the need for words. If our faces are without expression and our voices are flat, people are likely to think you are not listening or interested.

## 6.25 Thoughts cause feelings, feelings cause behavior

Mobile.

For younger, less skilled participants or a simpler, less time-consuming activity, plan any art/craft activity that lends itself to groupings of three. For older participants, a mobile offers an opportunity for sophistication and imagination. The goal for all skill levels is to have a lasting visual reminder of the power of association between thoughts, feelings, and behaviors/consequences. Tools: pliable wire, wire cutters, pliers, swivels.

### Objective

Make the connection between thoughts, feelings, and behavior and how they balance each other; understand the reasoning in cognitive restructuring.

### Implementation

1. Provide an example of a finished mobile for a visual support shortcut.

2. Discuss the relationship between thoughts, feelings, and behavior. For example, match the belief (thought) that hard work brings rewards, which in turn causes motivation (feeling) to work hard (behavior).

3. With paper and pen, make three headings:
   - thought
   - feeling
   - behavior.

   Draw on personal experience to make a list of matched thoughts, feelings, and consequent behaviors. For example, the teacher didn't believe that you didn't cause the fight with Joe. You think "it's not fair – unjust"; you feel "angry." What are you going to do about it?

   When identifying real-life associations, change the thoughts to see how that would have affected the outcome: "Well, I guess I shouldn't have thrown Joe's lunchbox over the fence – it would have made me mad too" (thought); you feel sorry (feeling); you apologize (behavior) and you are playing with Joe again after school.

   Back to the mobile: identify four groups of associated thoughts, feelings, and behavior that you've experienced. Represent each one with a symbol, a picture, or a word (a total of 12).

4. The pieces in the mobile might be:
   - painted on two cards – glue together, sandwiching a fishing swivel (or twisted metal loop) for attaching to the mobile
   - carved clay shapes – make hole or attach swivel/loop

- "wrapped" shapes – backed with attached fishing swivel.
- items with holes punched in them, simply tied
- paint symbols or words on tubes or pieces; glue metal swivels.

5. The larger mobile frame is constructed most simply from pliable wire, perhaps from a coathanger. The main frame will consist of a central post, the top of which will be either bent or have an attachment suitable for hanging, the bottom of which will form a loop through which two other cross-wires will branch out in four different directions.

6. Each cross-wire or branch will consist of a loop at each end from which will hang another (lower final) branch. Each and every branch is threaded through the loop above it and then twisted in the center for stability and to provide a loop for what hangs below it.

7. The final smaller branches, hanging from four different corners, will each have three loops (one at each end, one in the middle). From these loops, with string or lighter wired, hang the finished thought/feeling/behavior pieces.

**NOTE**
This is a time-consuming activity and will take a couple of sessions. However, it is not technically difficult and allows a lot of time for processing and discussion of real-life examples. Use the intervening time between sessions to recognize associated thoughts, feelings, and behaviors. Being able to question and change thoughts, feelings, and consequences is an important skill.

## 6.26 Fear, anxiety, confidence, esteem, and depression

Collage.

This activity can be broken up into a number of weeks. Each emotion can be the theme of several weeks. While each is important in its own right, the goal of the activity is to recognize the overlap and interaction of emotions – the chain effect and impact that unchecked emotions can have. Being able to make connections is important.

For example, Temple Grandin compares the emotions of individuals with Asperger's Syndrome to the unsophisticated emotional world of animals: "Fear is the main emotion." Yet fear can be manifested in anxiety, even generalized anxiety, and expressed through other behaviors and other emotions.

## Objective

Increase awareness of feelings, identify them verbally. Identify the relationship between the following feelings:

- fear
- anxiety
- confidence, esteem
- depression.

## Implementation

1. Represent each of the feelings through paint, paper, collage, ink, pens, torn pictures, words, pictures, colors, shapes, and so on. You may use one image for each emotion or a composite of images, textures, and colors. Allow time to explore what each feeling means to you. How does your body feel it? How does it affect your life? You may like to quantify the experience of feelings with a 1 to 10 score. The more you understand your feelings and their interdependence the better. Self-awareness is information. Information is power.

2. If you could paint the fear in your life, what would it look like? What does it feel like for you, what do you associate with it? Is it something you feel often in different areas of life? If you experience fear, what do you do to make yourself feel better? When you feel fear, do you sometimes get angry or avoid the situation or "act the clown"? (We all have coping mechanisms, sometimes helpful, sometimes not.) Ask these questions of each emotion, separately.

3. In the collage or image for depression, examine any experiences you may have of sadness, emptiness, crying, changes in sleeping patterns, always feeling tired or irritable, feeling things won't get better. How do you feel when you imagine your future? If you experience depression, what color does it look like to you? Does it have a shape? When can you escape the depression and what in your life makes you feel better? That's a lot to think about but it is important and these feelings often play into each other – they are very much connected.

4. Looking at the esteem image or collage, consider your strengths. In what areas do you feel you're not as good as you'd like to be? Do you compare yourself with others around you? If so, how do you compare? Do you have your own standards? If so, are you meeting your own standards? Sometimes, even if we feel we are meeting the standards we have set for ourselves, we don't feel confident when we're with other people. Perhaps you feel like a fish out of water, different or isolated, judged by others, not understood or valued by people around you. Do you sometimes avoid social situations because of a lack of confidence?

5.  As you're painting or tearing paper, stamping, and being creative, what thoughts come into your head? How much do these emotions overlap for you? Do the same situations bring about different emotions or is there one dominant emotion in most situations in your life? Are you uncomfortable with or unclear about your emotions or this exercise?

6.  Comparing the different feelings (and scores if necessary), are there strong similarities or differences? What would you change if you could? What could you change that would affect some or all of these emotions? How do you think that might change the balance between them?

7.  Is fear a dominant emotion for you as it is for Temple Grandin? Are fear and anxiety connected? Discuss and compare with group members. What do they fear? What is the nature and source and validity of fears? Do people with greater confidence have less fear and anxiety? This theme may be elaborated upon, depending on the participants and level of trust.

8.  For most people, strong self-esteem and confidence have the effect of reducing negative feelings. Do you think that might apply to you? If so, what concrete steps could you take toward raising self-esteem and confidence? If appropriate, construct a schedule of confidence-building experiences (see point 7 in exercise 6.28).

NOTE

It is relatively easy to say "I have low self-esteem" or "I am anxious." The goal of this exercise is to look below the surface and see how our feelings interact with each other and may have a domino effect. We can also modify feelings indirectly, through the domino effect. For example, if you gained confidence by winning a place on a school team, could that lessen anxiety in other areas?

## 6.27 Social anxiety and stress

Painting, expressive art, visualization, role play.

### Objective

Identify social anxiety.

### Implementation

1.  Draw a line down the middle of the page. On one side express how it feels to be in the most comfortable place in the world for you. Where is that? How often can you go there? Are you on your own or are other people with you? What does it look like? What does it feel like?

2.  On the other side of the page, express how you feel if you are standing in the middle of a room of people you don't know. It might be a party where you are expected to talk to others, it might be somewhere else. Do you feel comfortable? Do you fit in? How do you feel? What are you thinking? Imagine how your mind and body would be reacting and express that on the second side of the paper. Put feelings into words or paint and draw them.

3.  Compare the two sides and discuss differences in feelings.

4.  Stress for AS people comes from noise, tiredness, other people's expectations, and other people themselves. Emotions can shift in minutes from being an enjoyable experience to feelings of some form of distress. Many people with Asperger traits periodically experience tiredness from the effort of trying to meet other people's expectations, "pretending to be normal" as Liane Holliday Willey (1999) puts it. Identifying patterns in behavior allows prediction and anticipation.

    Do you feel stress with other people, after a long day, when at school, with lots of noise, in shopping centers? When did you last feel you had to "get away"? When did you feel trapped or overwhelmingly tired, perhaps to the point of tears or anger? Discuss the circumstances, conditions, feelings, and what led to the feelings and the consequences.

5.  Now, in imagination, go back to that same situation. Being cool and level headed, think about what you could have done to help yourself. Imagine what it would have been like if you had been able to have just five or ten minutes to yourself – privacy, being uninterrupted, no demands made of you. Where could you have found that space? Another room? The bathroom?

6.  Is it necessary to get upset in these situations, or argue with people? Role play a situation that is stressful for you, and practice different ways of saying "I need five minutes (or half an hour) to myself." Act out different possible responses to the following situations:

    -   At school, you are tired from playing sport at lunchtime; then back in class you help your friend Ben solve some problems with math; you still have to do your own math work and the teacher says she wants it all done before the end of the day; and then someone asks you to help carry some chairs up from the gym. You are physically tired, mentally tired, and stressed. What are good ways to get some stress relief in this situation? (Examples: places for quiet and privacy; visualization; relaxation exercises; explaining need for a few quiet minutes to a teacher.)

    -   You have just come home from school and are tired. You haven't had anything to eat since lunchtime but mom is busy and asks you to look after your little brother. Your homework needs to be done, your little brother is crying, and your sister is playing music very loudly. You suddenly feel overwhelmed with feelings and confusion and just want to scream. What are some of the things you can do to help yourself in this situation?

- What happens if you know something is likely to cause you stress but it simply has to be done? Break up the task into smaller steps or pieces and plan to spread the pieces out over a period of time. Allow or reward yourself with breaks. (I can lie down for 15 minutes then I will do the next bite-sized piece; paint the third wall; read another chapter.)

7.   If people put pressure on you to complete something, make a realistic plan and break it down into manageable parts. Be clear about your schedule and needs and then commit yourself to finishing each unit before taking the planned break. Ask for help. (I'll need two weeks; I'll need some assistance for the lifting and moving.)

Identify what is necessary for you to concentrate and focus and remain calm (a desk of my own where I know where everything is; quiet). Again, ask for help. Most people assume we all work the same way, think the same way, need the same things. Sometimes we need to simply and politely explain what we need to gain their cooperation. Practice making an appropriate request.

# 6.28 Anxiety: systematic desensitization

Systematic desensitization.

Used here to decrease anxiety, systematic desensitization is also very effective for dealing with: obsessive compulsive behavior (reduce the number of behaviors); phobias (increase length or degree of exposures, from imagined to real). For comprehensive "stress innoculation," combine with relaxation techniques.

## Objective

Systematic desensitization therapy for anxiety.

## Implementation
### COGNITIVE RESTRUCTURING

1.   What are your thoughts in a situation that causes you anxiety? Try to visualize yourself in a situation which causes great anxiety. It might be in a crowd of people, in a job interview, or approaching someone you'd like to know better. Close your eyes and see the surroundings, imagine every

detail as much as you can, feel your body, imagine the feelings. Let yourself sit in this imagined situation for a couple of minutes with your eyes closed.

2.  While you are imagining this situation and feeling the stress, what are your thoughts? Are you worried about the impression you make on other people there? Do you feel they are looking at you? Maybe you feel unattractive or uninteresting. What do you think you might be lacking? Maybe you're worried you'll be left standing in the middle of the room on your own all night, like an elephant at a mouse's party. Become aware of all the thoughts in this situation.

3.  Now, let's look logically at those thoughts. Open your eyes and write them down. Are you afraid of other people in a social situation? Are you anxious about what they might think of you? That you're not attractive? Go through your list and look at each thought – with the attitude of a research scientist. Where's the evidence? Where's the evidence that you are not attractive? That you have nothing interesting to say? That you stand out in the crowd?

4.  Let's look at possible alternative hypotheses. Perhaps people won't approach you because you look unfriendly, like you don't want to be there. Perhaps you're standing there with a face like you've been sucking lemons. Would you be keen to introduce yourself to someone like that? Perhaps you don't stand out in the crowd like an elephant at a mouse party. Perhaps people don't see you – you're like a mouse at an elephant's party. Indeed, most people think of themselves, what they look like, the impression they are making.

    Where's the evidence that you're not an interesting person? Who or what has made you think otherwise? You'd be interested in you, wouldn't you? On the other hand, some people think they are so interesting that they talk only about themselves – and other people want to get away because they don't want to spend their whole night listening to that.

5.  Most people like it when an interest is shown in them. How can you talk to people in ways that include them, show them you are interested, and make them happy to talk with you? (More on this in later activities.)

6.  A realistic awareness of yourself, your personal strengths, and unique qualities is important. Make a habit of questioning your own thoughts when you feel anxious. Remember, *just because you think it or believe it, doesn't mean it's true.*

## SYSTEMATIC DESENSITIZATION

7.  Write a list (a hierarchy) of five social situations. Begin with the least anxiety provoking situation – perhaps having lunch with a friend. End with the most anxiety provoking situation – perhaps going alone to a party. Between those extremes, you may have situations such as having

lunch with someone you don't know very well; initiating a conversation with someone you don't know at all; going into a room full of people you know and speaking to every one of them, one after the other. Set a goal for yourself that you will work through the list in the order that you have listed them.

8.  The first week, have lunch with your friend (or whatever the first item is). While you are doing this, enjoy it. Feel all the good things about it. Afterward, remember the good things and focus on them. Give yourself positive feedback.

9.  Visualize the next goal. Visualize the place, the situation, what the good things will be – a smile, wearing nice clothes, what you might talk about. When you come to do that goal, appreciate the good things while you are there, and remember them afterward.

10. Repeat the steps – focus on the pleasant parts of the experience, appreciate the good things, visualize or mentally rehearse the upcoming goal, focusing on anything pleasant and enjoyable. If you really don't feel you can go on to a step, repeat the preceding step, or modify it, taking it as close as you can to the step you are avoiding. It's about taking manageable steps, resting when we need to.

11. If social speaking is a problem, practice your skills in less anxiety provoking situations. Think of the worst possible scenario. If the worst possible scenario is making a speech in a party of 200 people, tone it down to smaller groups and less formal speaking. Perhaps a photograph of a crowd of people taped on the wall of an empty room might be the first place to start. Play a "tape" in your head imagining the best possible situation – people surprised at your genius, bowing in respect, bestowing honors. Take a friend with you and ask them to give you constructive feedback.

## 6.29 Relaxation strategies: social situations

Relaxation techniques.

### Objective

To decrease anxiety and relax in social situations.

### Implementation

1.  In exercise 6.28 it was suggested that you act like a scientist before making assumptions. (Where's the *evidence* that you aren't liked?) Of

course, it's difficult to be the hard-headed and logical scientist while your stomach is turning and your heart is racing. To get your body back under control, practice one of the relaxation exercises described in this book. It could be a progressive muscle relaxing exercise, although it's difficult in a room of people to clench and unclench all your face muscles without worrying people around you. You may relax with a visualization that you regularly practice in more comforting conditions.

2.  Practice bringing a peaceful visualization to the place that causes you anxiety (see activity 6.37). The first step is to practice being able to visualize the peaceful place in such detail and so often that you can recall it – and the feelings that come with it – almost instantly. It has been shown that thinking about something and visualizing it will cause the same reactions in your body as if you are actually there. If you can feel at home as easily in a party as sitting in your bedroom or on a beach, don't you think you'd feel more comfortable talking to people too?

3.  Another technique is to focus your mind on a tactile experience. At home take something that you enjoy the feeling of (piece of clay, wire spring) and play with it. Fill your mind with how it feels when you squash it or twist it, fill your eye with the color. It's difficult for the mind to focus equally on two things at the same time. If you are in a social situation and feeling anxious or an unwanted emotion, focus your mind's eye on the piece of clay, its color, how it feels to squash it, twist it, and so on. At the same time, breathe deeply and slowly. Sometimes in the attempt to suppress an overload of emotion there is a tendency to hold the breath, which makes the situation worse. Fill the lungs with new clean and calm energy.

4.  One of the quickest and most effective ways to relax (and stop an unwelcome surge of emotion in its tracks) is to breathe in deeply, counting slowly to ten, and then out again. Breathe in from your stomach, not just the top part of your body. Fill your whole body with oxygen. Repeat as often as necessary. Sometimes when we fear something or are trying to suppress emotion, we stop breathing without being aware of it. A brain full of oxygen is more in control than one that has been deprived.

Let's keep it in perspective. You're not running for president and world peace doesn't depend on the outcome of a social situation. What's the worst possible scenario? Will people throw tomatoes at you? Will you lose your job? Will a notice be put up in the public square announcing that you're an awful person? You are a unique individual with special strengths and attractive qualities – you will not show off your best qualities under all conditions but people who really matter will see them anyway and, as has been said, "There's always tomorrow."

You may wonder if it's worth the trouble. Isn't it easier to sit in front of the computer or television on a Saturday night than go to a party? Well, yes, it's easier. But have you sometimes thought, "Wow, I really didn't want to do this but I'm glad I made the effort – it's much better than I thought it would be." There's no guarantee that people will like us or we will enjoy ourselves or there will be a positive outcome if we put ourselves "out there," but the chances are much higher than if we spend every Saturday night avoiding our fears.

It helps to change expectations and yardstick for success. There may be another person there who is happier for speaking with you and feeling you were interested in what he or she had to say. Or, after three unsuccessful social outings, you may have a delightful time which made the first three efforts worthwhile. Lastly, as with most things, practice makes perfect. You have so much potential for a well-rounded and interesting life. Don't let your fears deprive you of that.

## Complex emotions

Individuals with Asperger's Syndrome typically have difficulty identifying and responding appropriately to complex emotions. Complex emotions can include sadness. It's easier to get angry than be sad. Anger is emitted in a burst that can get rid of the sad feelings at the same time. Understanding the underlying causes for emotions such as sadness and anger and being able to respond appropriately is important for self-regulation and positive choices.

### 6.30 Sadness

Expressive art, role play, interview.

#### Objective

Identify and express sadness appropriately.

#### Implementation

1. What is sadness? Discuss real-life examples of times when sadness has been felt, and situations that are likely to bring about sadness. When have you been sad? What did it feel like? How did you handle it? Have you seen other people sad? How did you know they were sad? How did you respond to it?

2. Paint sadness. What colors, lines, and textures do you think sadness would have if it was an image? You might like to paint one image for sadness (an animal, abstract shape, something) or a collage as in a mind

map, incorporating words. Explore what causes the sadness. Are there feelings of loss? Who or what is it that will be lost? What other feelings are around the feeling of sadness? (If necessary, close your eyes and remember a sad situation, bring back the feelings of sadness again, just to remember them.)

It's okay to feel sad. There are other things in your life that will support you in sad times. Incorporate words and images that show the things and people that support you when you are sad.

3.  Write a story about what sadness felt like for you. What brought it about and how did other people around you respond? What made you feel better?

4.  What do we do when other people are sad? Role play a sad situation and appropriate things to say. For example, a friend is moving away from your school and you will miss each other very much. You are both very sad. What can you say or do to make yourself and your friend feel better? Another example may be that a friend's grandmother has died. What are appropriate things to do or say in this situation?

5.  Speak about sadness with an adult who you know well. Ask them what has made them sad. What did they do when they felt sad? What made them feel better? If that situation happened again, what could you say or do to make them feel better?

6.  Compare notes in a group on this activity. What are appropriate responses to the sadness of other people?

## 6.31 Assertiveness, aggression, cooperation

Drama.

### Objective

Identify the difference between assertive and aggressive behavior.

### Implementation

1.  Read the following scenario:

    You have booked the tennis courts for a match on a Saturday afternoon. When you arrive the person who normally supervises the courts is not there. A couple of other people have taken your court and begun a game. You tell them you had the court booked but they just laugh and say they were there first.

2.  Use role play with a video camera and act out alternative ways of reacting to this situation. First, explore aggressive ways of reaction. What are the likely consequences? Then, explore assertive ways of behavior. What are the likely consequences?

3.  What is a real-life situation that has made you angry? How did you react? What was the outcome? What are other ways you could have reacted? What would appropriate assertive reactions have been?

4.  Discuss the difference between assertive and cooperative. Using the scenario above, role play different assertive and cooperative responses. What real-life situations have you experienced that could have used assertive or cooperative responses?

5.  In the role plays, some group members played the role of the "intruders," the people whose presence provoked the situation. What was their story? They may have been there because of a misunderstanding with regard to court bookings or they may have just believed if the court was empty they had the right to use it.

6.  Invite actors to make up their own stories about why they were at the court. After the role plays of aggressive, assertive, and cooperative responses, individuals who played the roles of the intruders discuss their emotional reactions to the different responses. What words, tone of voice, body language, or logic caused them to respond the way they did? (Review the video if necessary to see what triggered a response in the intruders.)

7.  What's the difference between assertiveness, aggression, and cooperation? When are appropriate times to use each one?

## Anger

Anger can be quiet, loud, positive, negative, justified or not, sometimes avoidable, sometimes not. Anger is usually the result of other emotions – from sadness to frustration, and very often fear. There is usually much more going on than the anger seen on the surface. Without understanding its nature, without self-management and regulation, anger can have very negative consequences. Basic approaches to managing anger positively include:

- relaxation skills

- cognitive skills

- assertiveness with self-regulation.

# 6.32 Anger management #1

Cognitive self-regulation.

## Objective

Explore feelings of anger; identify circumstances, physical reaction, and thoughts before, during, and after anger.

## Implementation

Identify physical feelings at times of anger – possibly warmth, tightness, shaking. Learn to recognize these feelings and examine your thoughts before you react with words. Feelings and thoughts and behavior trigger each other in a circle like wind, water, and a sailing boat. If you don't want to lose control, you, the sailor, should understand the effect they have on each other and bring them together in a way that gets you where you want to go.

1. Look at the feelings of anger. What makes you angry? (When things catch me by surprise; when things don't go as planned; when people are unfair to me; when I don't get my own way.) Who makes you angry? Are you angry a lot? Why control the anger? Does it fix the situation? Does anger stop it happening again? Does it get you what you want? Does it make you look good to people around you? Do you have more control and say things you really mean when you're angry? Let's look at some examples of what might have happened:

   - Ben hit me.
   - My sister is driving me crazy.
   - Someone scratched my favorite CD.
   - I'm not allowed to go to the movies.
   - My friend called me stupid.

2. Now let's look at the thoughts that go with the anger. What did you think about what happened?

   - Ben hit me.
   - I hate my sister.
   - This stuff always happens to things that are important to me.
   - My parents never let me do anything fun.
   - Everyone thinks I'm stupid.

3. Find three other possible explanations for what happened and your feelings.

   - Ben was told to hit me by aliens. Ben was angry at me too. Ben was angry because I broke his bike.

- My sister never gets into trouble. She's everyone's favorite. She doesn't like me.

- Someone broke into my house and scratched my CD because they don't like me. My mother accidentally scratched the CD when she was cleaning. It was scratched because I left it on the floor and I'm angry at myself.

- My parents hate me. They think I will be tired for school tomorrow. I really wanted to meet up with the new boy at school and be his friend.

- Everybody thinks I'm stupid because they're stupid. No one wants to be my friend. I am stupid.

4. Now think of other words that could explain the surge of feelings just after it happened: Frustration? Sadness? Embarrassment? Hurt? Anxiety? This is a powerful secret: *It's not what happens to you that makes you angry – it's what you think about what happens to you.* Not only that but the way you think about things gives you more or less power to change the situation.

5. Now let's look at the options for behavior:
   - Getting angry at Ben doesn't make things better – perhaps an apology for breaking his bike will.

   - Maybe your sister is everybody's favorite. You can't do much about that. Anger won't change it. But if she doesn't like you and that hurts you, perhaps you can do things to change that.

   - The scratched CD will cost money – anger won't change that. Perhaps making sure mom doesn't have the opportunity to scratch another one will stop it happening again. It's costing money but I've learned a lesson.

   - Maybe if I talk to my parents about how much I want to be friends with the new boy they will let me go to the movie with him. Maybe I can do something else with him on the weekend. Being angry with my parents isn't getting me what I want.

   - I hate that everyone thinks I'm stupid. I'm a bit worried because maybe I am stupid and they all see that. Am I stupid? Will I always be stupid? Why don't people like me? I feel so lonely sometimes. Maybe I should talk to someone I trust about this. Maybe they can help me find ways to understand if I am stupid and make the situation better.

We often jump to conclusions (one of the thinking traps) and assume the wrong thing. But our minds find it easier to "get angry quick" than to think about it. Being impulsive and getting angry is a dead-end street. Thinking about it helps to get control back and find ways out of a difficult situation.

Be careful of "all-or-nothing thinking." Be careful to avoid words like "always," "never," "everybody," and "nobody." Things are rarely as simple and absolute as they seem. Saying "nobody" and "everybody" is easy. But when you get down to the details, "nobody" and "everybody," "always" and "never" often just aren't right. Look deeper and find that there are many points of view, many explanations, and always more positive ways of handling something.

## 6.33 Anger management #2

Puppetry, drama, role play.

### Objective

Practice cognitive approach to anger management.

### Implementation

1. Recall a situation that has made you very angry and still makes you angry when you think about it. Perhaps someone did the wrong thing to you or you were blamed for something you didn't do. Explain the situation to the other people in the role play so that they can play the parts of the other people.

2. The first time you re-enact the scene, do so as closely as possible to the original scene. Say aloud the thoughts that are going through your head when the anger starts to rise again.

3. Write the thoughts down. The thoughts you had when you are angry are important but they might not be true. What are alternative thoughts you could have in response to this situation? Think of two and replay the scenario. What chain event does your changed thoughts put into place?

4. Now let's look at it backwards. Don't start with what made you angry. Start with the outcome of the original scenario. Perhaps you were made to look stupid or bad. What scenario would you have liked? What would be the best possible outcome in the circumstances?

5. Compromise: Life isn't always fair or clear. Sometimes there are situations where the other person is wrong and you are right, but you can do nothing about it. In these no-win situations, you may have to choose another course of action to bring about a better outcome than expression of anger.

- What are some situations over which you have little or no control?

- In some of the specific situations identified in the last question: if you can't change the situation, what can you do?

- Even if your thoughts don't change (I AM right, he IS wrong), could you change your behavior to change the outcome? What is the best outcome?

- When would it be appropriate to change your behavior even if you are right?

- When is being right the most important thing? Perhaps the long-term goal or outcome is more important than being right.

- How could you have changed your behavior for a better outcome, even if you are still angry?

6. Role play or act out with puppets. See how a change in you makes a change in the reaction of the other person – even if they're just acting.

## 6.34 Anger management #3

Visualization.

### Objective

Practice visualization to manage frustration and anger.

### Implementation

1. Think of something that makes you feel really good, or something that makes you laugh. It could be jumping in the pool or watching your friend do something really silly. Now close your eyes and imagine yourself back in that situation. Imagine, for example, a warm day, the color of the pool, what you are wearing, the sun on your back, running toward the water, leaping high and then coming down into the cold water. You are holding your breath and the cold water makes your skin tighten. You fall through the water until your feet hit the bottom. Then you push up from the bottom, through the bubbles. You burst through the surface of the water to take a deep breath. You are tingling all over, cold but happy, laughing. Sit and remember the feelings for a minute, how good it felt.

2. Change of scene. Spend some time reflecting on a situation that often ends up with feelings of anger. Close your eyes and remember an incident which has happened, perhaps many times with the same person. Remember what was said to make you angry. See the place where it is

happening, the other sounds and details around you. Now let yourself feel the anger that surges up inside you when this happens.

3.  Now, take back control. Calm yourself. Calm yourself by going back to the first scene – back to the pool, tingling, cold, and laughing. It's hard to stay mad while you feel like that. You are back in control, looking at what has happened with "cool, calm" thoughts instead of "hot and angry" thoughts. You are calm, you are in control, you are at the helm of your sailing boat. Now you can choose your direction, choose your behavior. Practice being able to switch off the angry feelings. If you practice it often enough, you will be able to use it when you need to control your anger.

## 6.35 Anger management #4

Expressive art, drama, puppetry.

### Objective

Manage frustration and anger through finding another perspective.

### Implementation

Another trigger for anger is often that we assume other people *should* see and act as we would. (Be careful of "should" words – they're similar to all-or-nothing words and are to be questioned.) Take as an example the last time you and a friend disagreed on something. Paint or write your perspective on the situation. Use words that made you feel emotional.

For the sake of the here and now, let's imagine you and your friend disagreed on whether or not you should go to the shore for a weekend. You love the shore – standing on the sand, letting the water roll around your feet – it makes you feel good and, as we know, emotions motivate our behavior.

Your friend likes the shore too but he is short of money at the moment. His worry about money is motivating him to argue for a much cheaper weekend. Now place yourself in the shoes (or chair) of your teacher who may have been sitting there. What would his or her perspective have been? Well, you didn't get good marks on science last semester – too many weekends at the shore. If his opinion was asked, he'd say staying home and studying would be a better way to go. *Each of us have different perspectives and, usually, different emotions to motivate us.*

Identify some situations that could make you feel angry. Who else is involved? Using art, drama, or puppets, imagine the emotions and reactions of the other people. Looking at the situation from their perspectives, what emotions are motivating them? Why are they behaving as they are? Is your anger necessary or useful? What would be a more useful response?

## Self-regulation

The following themes are ideas for self-reflection. Thoughts about each theme might be discussed in a group or individuals might role play real-life situations, different choices, and possible consequences:

- When does my behavior have negative effects for me or other people?
- When does my behavior have positive effects for me or other people?
- When do my thoughts control my behavior?
- When do I react without thinking?
- What choices do I have in how I react – and the possible consequences for each choice (specific and real-life examples).
- Some people and/or situations make me angry. What rules can I make for myself that could make those situations better for me?

Anxiety, worry, or anger are not just "all in the mind." They can actually change the chemicals in our body and hurt us physically.

A group discussion could include the following themes:

- In what situations do you "lose it" or have a "meltdown"?
- What are other words that can be used to describe how you feel?
- In your experience, what have been the outcomes and consequences of "losing it"?
- What sorts of things make you upset, frustrated?
- Are there times when you can predict beforehand that you may be upset/frustrated?
- If you can predict you may be upset in a situation or with a person, can you avoid it? What are your options and possible outcomes? (Be situation specific, draw from real-life dilemmas.)

- If you can't prevent getting upset, what can you do to calm yourself and regain some control?

## Self-regulating strategies

The students could choose to adopt the following strategies:

1. Read the relaxation strategies (activity 6.29).

2. Take yourself to your "special place" (activity 6.37).

   - Give yourself ten seconds to "find" your temper; breathe in, counting to ten. In your imagination, visualize finding your temper and regaining control.

   - In Guatemala, South America, "worry dolls" are sometimes used. Children tell their worries to dolls, the dolls are placed under the pillow, and the worries are taken away. Find a place of your own to put worries and negative feelings.

   - A creative activity can be to design and make a box, tin, container, or object of some kind that can be used as a place for safekeeping those emotions which can be overwhelming, hurtful, and not helpful. For example, sometimes anger and hurt might be better placed in a "box" until they can be dealt with more appropriately (better not to "resolve" things in a state of anger), or simply left there because if we can't do anything else about it it is better for them to be in a box than hurting and worrying us.

## 6.36 Self-regulation

Discussion, role play.

### Objective

Practice self-regulation with delayed gratification.

### Implementation

1. Controlling impulsive behavior is a common source of difficulty for the AS individual. Practicing delayed gratification is a cognitive skill that can be supported with logic, practiced and employed every day. Behavior is paired with expected consequences – consequences for "act now" and consequences for "act later." Although this is basically a cognitive

exercise, emotions are important because they provide the motivation to support the choice of behavior.

2. Role play versions of the following theme – integrate real-life analogies: Chris has a science assignment that is important for his end of semester grade. He knows the information and can write it up in one night – that will surely get him a B. On the other hand, if he doesn't go to the soccer match and goes to the library instead, he could get an A.

3. Role play the choice-making process out loud, including statements that form a triad – choice, outcome, and the feeling that the outcome is likely to produce. For example, "*If I forego the soccer game* and work harder on the project, *I will probably get an A*, maybe bringing me up enough to be admitted into the senior science classes, and that will *feel so good*, I'll be *happy and relieved* because I really would like to work with science."

4. Ben has just got $100 for his birthday from his generous grandmother. He has a choice between spending it at a theme park with his friends or beginning a savings account toward the new computer he wants. What are the different consequences of these two choices? What's the difference in feeling between the spend-it-now action and the save it/delayed gratification action? With that information, what choice would you make if you were Ben?

## Relaxation and imagery

People of all ages enjoy five minutes at the beginning or end of a session to relax with visual imagery. At the beginning of a session it can slow down group members whose minds might still be racing with the effort of getting there on time. At the end of a session it can be used to collect thoughts and leave a sense of completion, well-being, and positive thoughts.

The longer-term benefits are learning self-regulation techniques. Learned relaxation exercises can be used in the middle of the week to reduce stress or by some parents to stop a meltdown in its developing stages. This exercise is useful to practice slowing down and being conscious of thoughts and feelings rather than emotionally reacting to a situation. The following exercises are examples of relaxation and imagery exercises.

## o.37 Visualization

Relaxation, refocusing, and self-regulation.

### Objective

Visualize an image for quick recall, relaxation, and refocusing.

### Implementation

Participants sit in a comfortable position, not touching each other. Environment is quiet and cannot be interrupted. The facilitator reads the following story:

> *My special place*
> Close your eyes. Imagine you are in a beautiful part of the countryside. You look around you and the scenery is wonderful. The sun is shining and the colors are happy and beautiful. Breathe in deeply and smell the fresh air. The temperature is just right and the air feels wonderful on your skin. Your shoes are very comfortable so you decide to walk for a while.
>
> After you've walked for a while, enjoying the air and surroundings, you decide to sit and rest. You choose a nice shady spot next to some water and sit on a soft patch of grass. Some animals come by. They see you but aren't frightened. They eat near you and you sit and watch them quietly, still breathing deeply and enjoying the sights, sounds, and feelings. You feel so good that you decide to remember everything about this place and bring yourself back here in your mind whenever you want to feel as peaceful as this.
>
> Look around you. When you want to remember being in your special place, imagine looking at what you're seeing now. You feel very comfortable, not too hot and not too cool. When you want to be in your special place you will be able to see these things again and feel the good feelings. Take a minute of quiet to imagine and remember the details. Breathe slowly and deeply.
>
> Now, say goodbye to the animals and your special place. Breathe deeply and remember you can come back here anytime you want to. Close your eyes and breathe deeply. Now, as I count to five, open your eyes and come back to this room. One, two, three, four, five.

With practice, this image, along with the sensory associations, should be able to be recalled quickly (without the leading in process) and with ease. This is an invaluable tool for quick relaxing or refocusing.

☺

## 6.38 Progressive muscle relaxation

Systematic desensitization.

### Objective

Learn systematic and physical relaxing skills.

### Implementation

1. Stand up and give your body a gentle shake. Shake the arms, shake one leg at a time, roll your head. Now sit down comfortably on your chair, close your eyes, and follow my instructions. Feel your body, feel your breathing. I'm going to ask you to tighten the muscles in different parts of your body but I don't want you to squeeze hard – just enough to tighten the muscles under the skin before they relax again.

2. Let's start with your right foot and leg muscles. Clench the muscles a couple of times. Now give them a firm squeeze, not too tightly, and clench them while I count to five. One, two, three, four, five. Now slowly relax the muscles in your right foot and leg muscles. Totally relax them. Stay relaxed, breathe deeply, and feel the pleasure of the relaxation for a few seconds.

3. Now move to your left foot and leg muscles (repeat).

4. Now move to your right hand and arm. Open and close your right hand a couple of times. Now squeeze it into a fist, not too tightly, and hold it while I count to five. One, two, three, four, five. Now slowly relax the muscles in your right hand so that the hand falls open again, totally relaxed, like a rag doll. Stay relaxed, breathe deeply, and feel the pleasure of the relaxation for a few more seconds. (Wait ten seconds and proceed.)

5. Now squeeze your right arm, feeling the muscles in your right arm tighten, while I count to five. (Continue as in previous step.)

6. Buttocks, tummy, chest, shoulders (separately). Finally the face, jaw, eyebrows, scalp, clenching and stretching all the muscles, before releasing them, relaxed. Each part of the body is systematically relaxed.

7. Now feel the feelings of your whole body. Breathe in and then squeeze every part of your body, scanning quickly from the top of your body to the bottom of your body as you tighten the muscles and feel the feelings. Now, hold the tight muscles while I count to five and then release them again. Feel the pleasure as the feelings of relaxation wash over you. When you feel totally relaxed, open your eyes.

8. Practice this regularly at home, every day if possible.

# Yoga

Yoga is another form of relaxation. At the same time, it is an activity that can increase awareness of self and body. AS often presents problems with motor skills and coordination. There may be clumsiness or lack of awareness of space (inappropriate spatial relationships with other people). A multidimensional approach to support should include activities that offer opportunities to be aware of and in tune with the body. Yoga is ideal because it offers familiar routines that can be learned, is quiet and relaxing, and can integrate regulated breathing, which in itself is beneficial.

If the AS individual enjoys the basic exercises, classes with a qualified yoga teacher are recommended. The exercise below introduces yoga very simply. More sophisticated exercises focus on relaxed awareness and control of the body. They can be relaxing but some specific exercises also build strength and energy in non-stressful ways – useful for those AS individuals who feel disconnected with their bodies, have low muscle tone, and feel sluggish.

## 6.39 Yoga and breathing

Breathing techniques and movement.

### Objective

Extend relaxation skills.

### Implementation

### Breathing

1.  The diaphragm is the part of the chest, immediately under the middle of the rib cage, that expands with deep breaths. Locate the diaphragm with one hand and feel it rising and falling with the next step. It is important, when breathing properly, that the diaphragm actually expands and can be felt to expand.

2.  Breathe in, counting steadily to ten, then breathe out, counting steadily to ten. Feel the breath filling the body, from the bottom of the stomach, through the middle of the body, and up to the top of the chest. Then completely exhale, emptying the diaphragm and body of air.

3.  If there is discomfort or stress in the body, visualize clean air coming into the body and taking the discomfort and stress out of the body with the outward breath. Imagine the new air is bringing in a quiet energy. Perhaps it has a color, enabling the individual to "see" its effect. Another visual

image could be the ocean, bringing in waves which smoothly wash out again. Play relaxing music to assist in achieving a "flow" to breathing.

4.   Do this three to five times, whenever remembered. It is especially useful to regain concentration and control in stressful situations.

## Incorporating breathing with yoga

1.   Advanced students of yoga use poses that can be uncomfortable for new students. In the early stages, it is more important to be aware of the body yet comfortable. The goal is relaxation to enhance relaxation and that isn't going to happen with a cramp or uncomfortable pose. Students may lie on the floor, if space permits, or sit squarely in a position that suits them. If sitting, imagine a cord running through the center of the body, up through the head, as it might in a puppet. Now imagine the cord or string being pulled upward so that the whole body is pulled up straight. Using that image, find a comfortable but "straight and square" position.

2.   In that position, do slow and deep breathing, letting it flow into and out of the body. If thoughts are jumping around in the head, let them wash out of your mind with an outward breath. Concentrate on the flow, stretching the inner parts of the body with the flow of air.

3.   At the same time, be conscious of the different parts of the body and how the feelings in the body welcome the new breath, and release it easily and fully again. Be aware of the body sitting or lying, in that space, in that air, the temperature on the skin, the floor or chair supporting the body. The body is part of its surroundings. It is relaxed, comfortable, breathing, flowing – in – out.

4.   This alert/relaxed style of yoga and breathing can be integrated into walking activities. The individual may like to play music at the same time, or find an easy relaxed rhythm in the walking itself. This is an effective exercise for self-regulation of mood, being aware of the body, physically relaxing and clearing the mind.

## Depression

Common to all maturity levels is the need to understand the symptoms and character of depression and help individuals to develop strategies to help themselves or seek help when it is experienced. Without treatment it is likely to get worse or repeat again in the future.

Despite common fears, discussion of suicide does not increase its likelihood. Because of the common experience of depression and its association with suicide, support should include opportunities to be open about suicidal thoughts and feelings. *Any sign of suicidal thoughts and feelings should be taken seriously and addressed directly before the individual leaves the building.*

### 6.40 Depression #1

Handout – subject for discussion.

### Objective

Clarify the character of depression; pessimistic style of thinking; power of perspective.

## 6.40 Depression #1
## Handout

Depression may be the only condition or illness that we can have that denies our instinct to survive. With most illnesses, the mind and body fight to survive. In fact, if we trust and follow our instincts, we are sometimes able to find the resources inside our selves to heal.

Unfortunately, depression isn't like that. Depression can be like a vortex sucking you down into an emptiness with no end in sight. Perspective is lost and all-or-nothing thinking comes into play. Things will *never* change, *never* get better, life will *always* be unfair, and so on. Faulty beliefs are often the foundation for ongoing depression. In reality, given time, life will get better, things do change (nothing stays the same except change itself), and life, with its cycles, can be happy. But our happiness is determined by the way we think.

Let's put it this way. You are upset because you bought a new computer and the software that came with it did not include the office program you thought it would. You are very cranky and tell Tom, your flatmate, he can have the software that is of no use to you. But Tom plays around with the software and before you know it he is producing some great graphics, has started a business setting up other people's websites, and has made over $100,000 – all because he had another perspective on the same software package.

Our style of thinking plays into the perspective we take. Do you know someone who always sees the glass half empty while another who sees the same glass half full? Self-awareness – one of our greatest tools – not only helps us be more aware of what we have but our thoughts and attitude toward what we have.

Think about your life, your body, your mind, your family, friends, home, school, opportunities, future potential. Is your glass half full or half empty?

## 6.41 Depression #2

Collage, expressive art.

### Objective

Express feelings, thoughts, and associations with regard to depression.

### Implementation

If someone runs over your foot, you will probably feel pain. If someone runs over the feet of 20 people, all of those people will probably feel pain. But depression is more complicated than pain. Some people are more susceptible to depression than others. The same situation will affect different people differently – some may react with depression, others won't. Understanding the character of depression and a person's reaction to experiences in their life is important in managing it.

Use art to draw depression and associated feelings. If words can't be found, simply close eyes and "see" the sadness or emptiness or other feelings. Then scratch, paint, scribble whatever shapes and colors come to mind. Are there layers and hidden pockets? Feelings that are contradictory or not logical? The better these feelings are understood, the better they can be managed. What goes onto the paper does not have to make logical sense. You don't even have to find words for the feelings to acknowledge them and better understand them.

Always discuss feelings after an emotionally expressive activity. Despite long-held beliefs, catharsis is not always a good thing. Expressive art is best used as a tool to support discussion, conscious resolution, and empowering strategies.

## 6.42 Depression #3

Handout – subject for discussion.

### Objective

Understand depression in terms of an obsession. Can be used in conjunction with a schedule of concrete rewards and reinforcers to encourage changes to behavior.

## 6.42 Depression #3
## Handout

Depression is a type of obsession. An obsession is something we have an interest in, a relationship, something we spend a lot of time with. How can you have a relationship with depression? Depression is like a relationship where you're locked into yourself and excluding other people. If you've experienced depression, you will know it's like living with a bad or empty feeling. It can stop you from getting involved with anything or anyone else.

On Saturday night your friend Katie asks you to go to a party. If you're depressed you will probably be more interested in staying home with the sad and empty feelings than spending time with Katie. You don't think you can be happy. You don't want to be happy. You make no effort to be happy. You stay at home with the sad and empty feelings.

Why do you keep up your relationship with depression? While you're locked into yourself you don't connect with other people, the rest of life. It stops you from going out, from engaging in life. It tells you things will never get better (wrong!) and it judges you (I am awful, I'm not worthwhile). But it doesn't get you into anxiety-provoking situations. It kills the pain because it takes you out of feeling and out of life, it keeps you empty, without energy.

What purpose does depression serve you? Why would you want to stay with it? It dumbs you down, numbs you down, right? You don't have to get anxious, you can just be empty and avoid life – maybe for years.

Wait! For years?

Some people stay depressed for years. Is anxiety that bad? With the right support and approach it can be a firewall to go through. Who knows what's on the other side of the wall or what the future could bring. Anxiety won't kill you. But depression might.

Discuss what depression does to you. It would take courage to engage in life again. If you are depressed, what are some of the things you can do, personal strengths you can use or people you can speak with to help you?

## 6.43 Interests and obsessions

Box, altered book.

### Objective

Become aware of the nature of interests and obsessions, the degree to which they dominate time.

### Implementation

Obsessions can be great. They teach us new things, provide an interest to fill leisure hours, and we can become experts in something that we really like. But when does an obsession cross the line to become unhealthy?

ACTIVITY #1 NOW

1.  Make a three-dimensional collage out of a box or altered book (old book, cut hole/s out of pages which are then glued together, effectively forming a box between the book covers).

2.  On the outside – use fabric, paper, pictures, symbols, photos, paint, pens, found objects, etc. to represent interests and their effect on your life. Include the wonderful, useful, or positive things about your interests. Also include the less wonderful things (cost, time).

3.  On the inside of the box – use fabric, paper, pictures, symbols, photos, paint, pens, found objects, etc. to illustrate and represent your potential, your dreams – what you could do if you had the time and money, what you'd like to do one day or may never do but dream about. Potential is exciting. It is an important part of you even if it remains undeveloped, unfinished, unrealized.

4.  Each of us is unique, with unique skills, opportunities, and potential. Unfortunately, what we do with our potential will be limited by time. Giving time to anything takes time from other things. Being responsible for ourselves includes being responsible for the way we spend our time.

Look at the finished box and draw your own conclusions. Are you spending so much time in just one or two areas that there is an imbalance? What would you like to spend more time doing? Where might you spend less time to make time for that? Can you balance your life a little to include more of the things inside the box that are waiting to come out and grow?

ACTIVITY #2 TAKING YOUR INTEREST INTO THE FUTURE

1.  Where would you like to be in five years' time? In ten years' time? Would you like to be using your special interests in your work? What sort of work would you like to do? Brainstorm/spider map ideas about

combining your interests with work. From that write a list of interesting jobs that are connected in some way to your interests and skills.

2.   Homework: Do research on the jobs on the list – the internet, library, guidance officer. Talk to people with similar interests or who are already working in the area. What suggestions do they have? Be as concrete and as definitive as possible in describing job possibilities, the advantages, disadvantages, personal interest, requirements. Would you be required to do specialized study and are you prepared to do that? How would it fit in with other plans you may have for the future? If you followed this path, would you make the amount of money you'd like to earn?

3.   Given the information you now have, what direction would you like to go in with your interest? At this stage, what is your ultimate goal or achievement in this area? (Interests and circumstances may change.) What do you have to do, in concrete steps, to reach the final goal? How can you reward yourself for small steps in that direction? Who might mentor or support you? What are the weakest links?

# A happy and resilient future

**Learn and enjoy learning**
Enjoyment of learning adds to resilience. Making activities interesting, and stimulating new interests will contribute to positive development.

## 6.44 A happy and resilient future #1
Handout – subject for discussion.

### Objective
Identify innate signature strengths.

## 6.44 A happy and resilient future #1
## Handout

We assume that if we remove the things in our life that make us unhappy, happiness will automatically be there.

Wrong. Things will always come into our lives to make us unhappy. It might be stubbing a toe, finding that color blindness will stop a dream to become a pilot or the death of someone close. We cannot stop disruptive things from happening, and even if we could happiness cannot be guaranteed. We have all met people who have everything and should be happy but they're not. If you want to build a happy life for yourself there are a couple of things you can do to help.

1.  The first is to identify what will make you happy and make plans to include those things in your life. Imagine being lost late at night because you weren't following a map and you end up miles from anywhere – not a happy situation. Potential is a wonderful thing but it's much better when it gets you where you want to go. You need to be at the end of the right road, or at least in the right direction to the right destination. Do you know what the right direction would be for you to be happy? Don't let the wind blow you around and hope the wind blows you in the right direction. Think about it, make goals, take action.

2.  The second thing you can do to make a happy life is to find ways to bounce back from the unhappy events that inevitably happen in our lives – develop *resilience*. We can take action to become more resilient and more adaptive when faced with disruptions, disappointments, and crises.

    Activity 6.17 is an exercise to identify personal strengths. Review your personal strengths, using the list in Appendix 1. These are personal strengths that are very useful in building a happy life (Peterson and Seligman 2004). Which five do you think you are strongest in?

3.  Identify your five signature strengths and then imagine and discuss how they could be applied to problems in your life now. In what ways can these strengths help you recover from difficult experiences?

4.  Go beyond your signature strengths. What other qualities on the list do you think would be useful to have? How would you apply them? What can you do to make those skills stronger?

## 6.45 A happy and resilient future #2

Painting, collage.

### Objective

Identify what makes you happy now; what might make you happy in the future?

### Implementation

Identify what makes you happy now and what you think would make you happy in the future. Envisage what a happy future would look like and then express that with paint or a collage. In this activity you might like to use the quality of "playfulness and humor" – there are no rules with imagination. You are an original and unique individual – use that in designing a life for yourself. Have fun and be inventive. Be expansive and innovative in thinking about the possibilities.

## 6.46 A happy and resilient future #3

Keyring, bracelet reminder.

### Objective

Identify five signature strengths and make a keepsake as a reminder.

### Implementation

1.  From the list in Appendix 1, identify five signature strengths. You may like to show the list to friends, family, and teachers and ask them which they see as your five greatest strengths.

2.  Discuss in your group how those strengths can give you resilience in times of trouble. How can they be applied to real-life situations?

3.  Make a symbol or word for each of the strengths.

4.  Put the symbols on pieces of wrapped card or oven baked clay tiles. Put them on a keyring or bracelet to carry with you to remind you of your signature strengths – and resilience.

## 6.47 Making amulets

Mixed media.

Amulets are traditional symbols of protection that people carried with them in countries such as Egypt, Thailand, Italy and in many Indian tribes. The custom is thousands of years old and the amulets can take the form of written wishes, symbols of lizards and turtles, Buddha and other things. They're usually carried around the neck.

1.    From the list in Appendix 1, choose a strength that you have that could protect you in difficult times.

2.    Write the strength as a word or draw a symbol of it. You may wish to write it on a strip of paper and then roll and glue the paper into a "bead" with the word hidden inside. You may wish to paint the symbol on a small stone or carve it into clay.

3.    When the symbol of your signature strength has been completed, protect it with a small wire cage (twist wire into a spiral "cage" with pliers, twisting or adding links for attachment) or a leather pouch (a project in itself). Attach the wire cage or the leather pouch to a cord that will hang around the neck. Carry this symbol of your strength with you to remind you of its protective powers.

# Puppets

Puppets serve a multitude of purposes. *Designing and making puppets* employs creative, imaginative, sequential processing; sensory integration, motor skills, coordination and sequencing, holistic thinking.

*Giving a performance* involves conceptual thinking, teamwork, sensory integration (words, music, texture, lights, etc.), scriptwriting, and sequencing.

*Using puppets* allows the participant to step back and see actions, interactions, and reactions from a detached perspective, learning through watching, modeling, and projecting the self. Other benefits include the following:

- Different issues can be explored with a minimum of risk (safety, negative outcomes).

- Encouragement of participation from quiet members who can speak through the puppets, lessening the egocentricity that often dominates interactions with more outgoing members.
    Opportunities to practice organization and teamwork, cooperation

and coordination with others – and coordination of other puppets on a "stage."

- Brainstorming, cartooning, scriptwriting, rehearsing, role playing, and videotaping are varieties of the same theme – repetition in practicing and learning skills.

- Puppets can be personalized or made into caricatures and actions exaggerated – expressive and projective opportunities.

- Conversation skills can be practiced in novel ways, adding humor, imagination, non-conventional approaches; also taking turns, topic maintenance, reciprocity.

- Narrative skills are enhanced – the process of telling stories (cohesion, sequence) and the tone with which they're told (animation, variety of tone, appropriate volume, rhythm); rehearsal, practice, and familiarity may improve synchrony.

- An AS trait is to avoid eye contact because of the problems with sensory overload. Puppets don't require eye contact which allows for more concentration, focus, and learning than role plays with real people.

- The "beginning" and "end" of a script and performance provide a structure that is pleasing to the AS desire for control and completion. They are not "left hanging," not knowing where to go or what to say next.

- Puppets put more fun into the learning experience – with increased enjoyment, receptivity, and retention.

Puppets are reasonably cheap to buy. However, making them offer opportunities for genuine expression and originality, employment of motor skills, appreciation of individuality and wit. There are many useful books describing techniques for puppet making. A highly recommended book is *Marionettes: How to Make Them and Work Them*, by Helen Fling (1973). It offers comprehensive information simply and is excellent value. A more accessible source is the website www.puppetbuilder.com which also has a list of recommended books.

## 6.48 Making puppets: me and other people

Three-dimensional collage, mixed media.

### Objective

- The objective of this exercise is to represent different people – family, friends, figments of imagination – through sculpture, puppets, three-dimensional objects.

- The way that people are represented (expression, clothing, props) is in itself important and could be the subject for further exploration.

- The way that people are discussed during the creative process is worthy of note.

- After the objects have been made, they can be kept for future reference and exercises to illustrate family dynamics, social situations, and so on.

### Implementation

- Puppets can be glove puppets, hanging puppets (marionettes), rod puppets.

- Heads might be attached to wire covered bodies or to springs or pieces of card/clay linked together for a dangling puppet body. Foam, cloth, and paper are some of the materials that can be used for bodies.

- Different techniques and materials – and few "rules" – endless potential for truly original puppets. Some heads, bodies, and unfinished puppets can be provided as a visual explanation for construction yet leaving the finished product open to imagination.

- Clay head: Take a piece of Fimo, Premo, or similar clay to be oven baked. Roll it into a ball. Now squish it into a shape. If we know the head belongs to Dad, we don't have to make it look like Dad. Make a hole to insert wire or stick after baking. After baking, paint the face, apply hair (paint, fabric fringe, craft "hair," hair cut from a dog, twisted wire). Insert the wire/stick body. Assemble legs and arms which have been shaped and baked at the same time. Dress, drape, attach to a base (clay, wood) which can be moved around the stage, or a rod which can be held.

#### ROD PUPPET

This puppet is built around a stick or rod. It can be built up, wrapped, or covered like a three-dimensional collage. Materials might include a clay or ball head, or a framework covered in soft, flexible materials (paper, cloth, foam).

## HAND PUPPET

The simplest puppets can be made by cutting fingers off gloves and decorating them. A hand puppet will use a glove, tube, or sock for a base. Eyes, features, clothes, and character can be added through paint, other materials, found objects. It might take on the shape of the hand or form might be added with padding and foam.

## STANDING PUPPET

This is useful for representing a character, whether or not it moved around a "stage." It can also be treated as a three-dimensional collage. Because it stands up it must have a base which won't topple and will hold the body – a block of wood, a base of baked clay, a circle of heavy metal, an upside down flowerpot, heavy candle, anything solid of interesting shape and right size that won't be tipped easily.

The body must also be support-ive – wood, baked clay, wrapped card, a spring, found object. The body might be an extension of the base or can be glued to the base, stuck in the base, or bound to the base (and the head) with a stick, wrapping wire or fabric, wire frame, clay core. The head can be an exten-sion of the body or an entirely differ-ent material – clay, cardboard, stamped, painted, molded, squished or delicately formed, wrapped in fabric or a raw wooden ball – and decorated with any array of painted or found objects to add individuality and character (Figure 6.1).

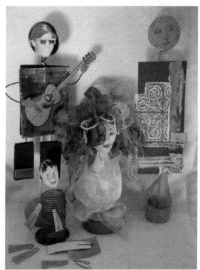

*Figure 6.1 Standing puppets: characters*

## HANGING PUPPET

It can be used as a marionette or hung from any number of things. Use the same principles as above but have limbs in flexible materials, linked pieces, or fabric sausages and attach them with split-rings, pieces of fabric, ribbons, and so on.

Interesting bits and pieces, including glass eyes, are sold by sports shops as materials used to make lures. A coat of paint or glued paper will transform many boring pieces found in a hardware store or the kitchen into an amazing array of bases, bodies, and heads. Praise should be given for initiative, originality, wit, flexible thinking, and innovative ideas.

> Fun and imagination are strengths that add to resilience. Being commended for originality adds to self-concept. Having fun in a group is one of the ultimate goals of social skill groups.

## 6.49 Me and my family #1

Three-dimensional collage, mixed media.

### Objective

Identify individual in context of family relationships.

### Implementation

1.   Using clay, make figures to represent different members of your family or significant others in your life, or use figures from activity 6.48.

2.   Paint and decorate in ways that describe the character of the person as you know them. Perhaps they are sweet to everyone outside the house, but the relationship with you is volatile. Thinking back to symbolism, how can different characters be represented? Would stripes indicate different sides of the character? Would pink describe someone in your family? You may wish to cover someone with tiny musical notes or torn up strips of colored paper. Drape the bodies with a scrap of fabric, paper, or found objects. Faces might be simple balls of clay with eyes and mouths drawn on them (practice on paper first) or stamped with a face stamp or shaped with your fingers (most fun and lots of room for caricature). Three-dimensional characters are a wonderful opportunity to be extremely creative. Don't forget the family pets.

3.   Now that your figures have been completed, arrange them in a family scene. Who is the central figure in your family? Who has the most influence on everybody else? Put them in the middle and arrange other people around them according to how much influence and what kind of connection they have.

## 6.50 Me and my family #2

Genogram.

### Objective

Identify individual in context of family relationships; build awareness of support network.

## Implementation

1.  Develop a visual picture of your extended family. Use many different colors of pens and paint. In light pencil, before you start, draw lines on large pieces of paper to represent generation "levels."

2.  Put yourself in the center of the bottom level. From that point, develop the genogram like a map, representing older generations in higher levels, connecting people with lines that describe their relationship. Make a connecting line between you and any siblings on the same row. Males should be represented by one shape (usually a square but you can be different) and females by another shape (usually a circle).

3.  On the level above you, illustrate the generation older than you – parents, and their associated siblings. If uncles and aunts have children, represent them on your level with different shapes.

4.  Continue this process to include as many people as you have knowledge of.

5.  Now concentrate on the types of relationships that are between different people. You can make lines between yourself and other people in the family, using colors or lines and/or words to describe your relationships, their influence, feelings about those people. Focus on positive stories – how have people been helpful to you? What good memories do you have of them? Who continues to be a supportive influence?

6.  Around each person make other associations. To the best of your knowledge, what was their home and community like? Their family relationships? Who and what influenced them? What influence do you think that may have had on the family and people around them?

7.  If you had a relationship with them, what was it like? What were their personalities like? What other information is significant in their relationship with you? Point out the reason to participants for focusing on positive relationships – these are the relationships (even if they are in the past) that help build a resilient character in the family.

8.  If conditions permit, or homework can be given, write out a thoughtful summary of how the family in its parts or as a whole has provided and continues to provide positive influence and support.

9.  Identify qualities, strengths, memories or cultural experiences that can be drawn from the genogram and used as key words or a motto to be incorporated in a family crest or shield (two- or three-dimensional – good activity using clay).

## Values

Individuals with AS typically have a narrow understanding of emotions – their own and other people's. Earlier exercises have paired emotions with thoughts and behavior. Cognitive restructuring is an excellent support for self-regulation and managing emotions – by balancing emotional reaction (or over-reaction) through questioning the validity of thoughts. However, depending on the skill level, cognitive restructuring may be taken further, into the area of beliefs and values in which our thoughts are grounded.

As an example, if there is distress because "Holly isn't talking to me – I thought she was my friend," it may be appropriate to question the associated values. "Why do you think Holly is your friend?" "What do you expect from friendship?" "Do you have rules for friendship and Holly has broken them?" "What if Holly doesn't have the same rules?" "What if Holly wasn't aware that you considered her a friend?"

The following activities relate in different ways to values. Positive Psychology considers ability to think critically, have an open mind, and make appropriate judgments as supporting resilience. Evaluative thinking and ability to make objective judgments can be problematic for the AS individual. Clarifying values helps guide thoughts, judgments, and choices. Acknowledging others' values helps understand differences and leads the way to cooperation.

Personal values also provide another source of strength for a "meaningful" and engaging life, which in turn offers resilience and protects against depressive tendencies.

*Improvised drama, discussion, mind maps*

The following themes may be used for discussion:

1. What makes a person "good" or "great"?

2. Who do you admire and why?

3. What are values and what do they mean to you?

4. What do you think are good values to have?

5. What purpose do values have?

6. Where do values come from and can they be changed?

7. How can having a set of values affect your life in the short term and the long term?

8. What rules would you make if you were the President of the United States?

9. What would a "perfect world" be like?

10. What would you like to achieve in your life, more than anything?

11. If you could do something over again, what would it be?

## 6.51 Values #1: goal setting

Discussion.

### Objective

Increase awareness of values and their impact on direction and motivation. Positive development is initiated and guided by goals, consciously or subconsciously. A weak link in the goal-setting process for an AS individual is often lack of self-awareness and how personal values can impact on aspirations. Discuss the following questions leaving the conclusions open:

1. What aspirations do you have for yourself? Do you have a picture in your head of where you'd like to be or what you'd like to do in the future?

2. What is most attractive about this picture? Why are these goals important to you?

3. Have you set yourself goals (with definite steps) to reach those aspirations? Do you have a timeline?

4. What is most important to you (interests, values, how you like to spend your time, with whom you like to spend time, what you would like to achieve)? How do these things fit with your goals?

5. Is there anything you'd like to avoid as much as possible?

Realistic assessment and consequences:

6. Do you have what you need to achieve your goals?

7. What strengths do you have to help you achieve them?

8. What do you need to learn or acquire?

9. How realistic is that? What steps do you need to follow?

10. What do you think could stop you from reaching your goals?

11. How can specific disadvantages and difficulties be overcome?

12. Are you lacking in confidence? Explore the validity of the lack of confidence.

13. Do you have enough control to make necessary changes? If you feel you don't have control, how valid is your belief? Where can you be effective in making positive changes for yourself?

14. Setting goals and the process of achieving them will be restricted by the picture we see for ourselves. But sometimes our goals can't be reached because of external factors. How could some of the following interfere with your goals and how can you anticipate and manage them?

- time
- support or lack of support from other people and your environment
- other people's expectations
- stress.

## Rules

Planning and building a life that fulfills potential and is resilient in the face of disappointment requires awareness of values and motivation for choices made. If taught early in life, individuals with AS will learn the "rules" and adhere to them without question. The problem is that sometimes rules have to change, are inappropriate. The resilient person is flexible and adapts to changing situations while relying on their own strengths and standards. Temple Grandin (1999) has broken the logic of rules into four categories:

- really bad things (murder)
- courtesy rules (manners)
- illegal but not bad (some laws were made to be broken)
- sins of the system (varying between different systems).

These rules are externally imposed and support society. While the individual may abide by them, they do not provide answers when personal situations and dilemmas arise (a partner is unfaithful; a friend is doing something wrong and asks for it be to kept secret). There will be times when personal internal values and standards need to be constructed and referred to.

## 6.52 Values #2: rules

Discussion.

### Objective

Social interaction, moral reasoning, hypothetical, abstract, and conceptual thinking.

### Implementation

Discuss the following questions – leaving the conclusions open:

1. When, in your life, have you not known what the rules are?
2. When do the rules seem silly or wrong or don't fit your situation?
3. When do rules not work? What should you do when rules don't work?
4. Why have rules? What's important enough for rules?
5. What rules work for you? What rules don't?
6. What rules would you make for yourself? Why?

> **Citizenship, duty, teamwork, loyalty**
> Citizenship, duty, teamwork, and loyalty are strengths that enhance resilience.

## 6.53 Values #3: teamwork and citizenship

Discussion.

### Objective

Build awareness of social interaction and moral reasoning.

### Implementation

What are citizenship, duty, teamwork, and loyalty? Discuss the following questions:

1. How important are citizenship, duty, teamwork, and loyalty? Why?
2. Looking at teamwork, what are the qualities of a good team? What are the qualities of good leadership?
3. Would you be a good leader? What are three characteristics about yourself that would make you a good leader? What are three

characteristics about yourself that may need to be modified for you to be a better leader?

4. Would you be a good team member? What are three characteristics about yourself that would make you a good team member? What are three characteristics about yourself that may need to be modified for you to be a better team member?

5. What are examples of loyalty? When is it not a good thing? Under what circumstances would you stop being loyal to someone?

6. Discuss citizenship with examples of the advantages, disadvantages, and values connected to citizenship.

7. Discuss duty with examples of the advantages and disadvantages, and when it is a good thing or bad thing.

8. Are citizenship, duty, teamwork, and loyalty based on social values or personal values? (Are you a good citizen because your society expects it or because you want to be a good citizen?)

These questions could be followed by a discussion about why citizenship, duty, teamwork, and loyalty are strengths that enhance resilience. How could each of them give you strength in difficult situations?

## 6.54 Values #4: shades of gray

Group activity, discussion.

### Objective

Social interaction, moral reasoning, hypothetical, abstract, and conceptual thinking, prioritizing, categorizing, connectedness.

### Implementation

In a discussion with the group, write down morally questionable situations that are morally "bad" – from mildly bad to the worst behaviors. They might include keeping secrets, not reporting income to the IRS, taking the car without asking permission, telling lies, selling drugs, being cruel to animals, driving while drunk and killing someone.

1. Discuss each situation, to what degree it is "bad," whether it could ever not be "bad," our moral obligations, potential consequences of a world with no moral values, whether we should set our own values or they should be set for us, and so on.

2. Cut the words up (or symbols representing them) and then put them in some sort of order, from "least" to "worst." Do different group members move the words into different positions? Why?

3. Introduce some hypothetical situations such as situations when a wrong behavior might be made right, or at least acceptable, and perhaps move up the list. Can examples be found to dispute the position of different behaviors? (Is telling lies always bad? Could stealing ever be excused?)

The goal of activity 6.54 is to break down concrete thinking and introduce the idea that there are gradations in moral behavior and different consequences, often depending on context; practicing non-concrete discussion where facts are debatable, respecting and integrating the opinions and points of view of others; and thinking of moral issues from a conceptual rather than a rule perspective.

A variation on activity 6.54 is to focus on "good" behaviors – to what degree are we obligated to other people and why (sending birthday cards, helping strangers), whether behaviors should be accepted because of social rules (why is it a social rule not to call people by their first name or ask how much people earn?), and who do social rules benefit? What motivates "good" behaviors and to what degree should we make self-sacrifices for others?

Gauging and enhancing a sense of *internal control and connectedness*. Can we make a difference in our world? How? Should we try? If appropriate, from this small discussion goals might be set and met, individually or collectively. For example, a love of animals might lead one or two group members approaching local shelters for volunteer work.

## 6.55 Values #5: personal

Group activity and discussion, scriptwriting, role play, drama.

### Objective

Establish personal reasons for making choices; effect and outcome possibilities.

### Implementation

1. As a group, write a script about the unresolved personal dilemma of a group member (drawn from experience). Example: Someone you've always admired invites you to the Bahamas for a weekend. You have a

boyfriend or girlfriend who would be upset if they knew about it. Maybe he or she doesn't need to know.

2.  In the script, set up the scenario with the main actor and relevant people who are involved or may be affected (giving a face to those who may not be in attendance in real life). Give the main actor three or more possible choices of behavior. Example: Yes, no, not this weekend, next weekend. Is my boyfriend/girlfriend invited? Not this year, maybe next winter.

3.  Act and improvise possible outcomes from the choices made. Each choice may be acted out a number of times, with different people in different roles, giving different perspectives (including those who may be involved/affected).

4.  Each group member gives each choice a rating from one to ten on how "right" or "wrong" they would evaluate each choice, giving reasons for their rating. Discuss.

5.  Considering everybody's perspectives and feelings, what would be the best possible outcome?

6.  Would different people in the group make different choices? Is there only one right way of doing something?

7.  What is a dilemma common to members of the group (perhaps wondering what to do about a friend using drugs)? Try to resolve the dilemma as a group. Compare different perspectives and values. Perhaps role play hypothetical conversations with the friend. Giving a voice to other "players" in the drama gives more credence to their influence. Actors representing other players may also have their personal perspectives to contribute. Examples of other themes may be whether or not to intervene when a school bully picks on someone else; or what to do when a student knows cheating is happening in an exam.

## Transitions

Transitions are pivotal points in every adolescent and young person's life, with or without Asperger's Syndrome. Because there is a step from the familiar into the unknown, the predominant feeling is often loss, grief over the loss, fear about the unknown, and doubts about whether or if the changes can be managed.

## 6.56 Experiencing transition

Art, discussion.

### *Objective*

Clarify the different aspects of a transition.

### *Implementation*

1.  Do a painting, drawing, or collage to identify a current area of change or transition, and the feelings about that change. The group facilitator may initiate some discussion about transitions, making note about the normality of changes throughout life, and in particular as individuals move from childhood toward maturity. Examples of change and transitions may be concrete (getting a driver's license, going to college) or they may be more emotional and difficult to express (increased responsibility with independence and perhaps living away from home, changing feelings towards friends of the opposite sex).

2.  Identify the emotions associated with a particular transition – the immediate and obvious emotions, and those that may be underlying them (if anger is involved, what might be provoking the anger and how is it managed?).

3.  Make a list of those things that the individual feels they are losing – concrete (friends, familiar surroundings) and associated losses (confidence, control). What is becoming less important, changing or finishing?

4.  With experiences of change and loss, other doors open. Make a list of the new opportunities, the things that are or may be gained, what is becoming increasingly important or beginning?

5.  Go back to Personal story #1: life map (6.2). "Ups" and "downs" of life are graphically represented in a sort of timeline. Use this exercise to remember the feelings around those events, what helped at the time (coping mechanisms, helpful people, own skills), and outcomes. Acknowledge the personal growth that has come out of change and the potential for positive, sometimes surprising, outcomes. New friends may have been made along the way, new interests developed, and good memories made. How can some of the lessons learned from this exercise be applied to help changes being made at the present time?

## Self-awareness

Self-awareness provides the basic foundation from which changes can be made.

Creative activities and interventions can be designed to develop self-awareness – strengths, weaknesses, perceptions, reactions, thoughts, and beliefs about people and situations, and a supportive context in which to challenge any unrealistic thoughts and beliefs. It is through these exercises that goals, motivations, tasks, and meaning emerge – all of which can play a part in building resilience.

Cognitive behavioral therapy or changing the way we think is a most effective way to change behavior. Another approach is to change the behavior which will produce a change in outcome – and thoughts about the behavior will change as a consequence. For example, if an adolescent has difficulty changing thoughts, of anger toward a classmate, a different behavior such as including the person in an invitation to a game or the movies may produce a friendlier experience with them, and consequently changed thoughts about them.

A group is useful for changing patterns of thinking (cognitive behavioral therapy, CBT) because when experiences are shared often other group members can contribute to a discussion of alternative ways of thinking and being, check the reality of thoughts, and support efforts to change behavior. Again, self-awareness plays an important role in effective CBT treatment. Creative therapies help stimulate new ways of thinking about ourselves and our roles rather than reiterating the "old stories."

In conclusion of this chapter, self-awareness is a work in progress, in concert with life itself. Creative expressive activities cannot be overestimated in their value for increasing self-awareness and responsibility.

# CHAPTER 7

# Social difficulties and connecting with the world

By adolescence, traits of Asperger's Syndrome are often modified to the degree that they are hardly noticeable. But underlying modes of thinking remain the same and support may be needed for new demands – building adult friendships, working relationships, and intimate partnerships, getting a quote, a refund for a defective toaster, asking for help, and being wary of unscrupulous behavior of others. Group support should encompass:

- anticipation, discussion, and practice of possible and actual social scenarios
- formal education with regard to the value of connectedness with others for a positive life (reiterated in activities, exercises, discussions)
- informal support, using the group to model and build genuine friendships, cooperation, teamwork and sincere interest in each other encouraged, and being a valued contributing member of a community.

Useful activities and discussions can focus on themes such as:

- school
- home, with family
- friends and social groups.

**Curiosity/interest in the world**

Two of the strengths purported to enhance resilience are curiosity and interest in the world. The importance of being connected to people has been discussed and appropriate activities suggested. Being connected to organizations, work, goals, and causes provides a resilient satisfaction and growth.

## 7.1 Connections in my life

Genogram, painting, collage.

### Objective

Identify levels of relationships, support network, character of relationships.

### Implementation

1. Do a collage/painting that illustrates people in your life. It may be:
   - a genogram (described in activity 6.50)
   - a mandala (with the most important people in the middle, less important toward the edges of the paper)
   - a tree (the most important people in the trunk, less important people on branches that may splinter, fall off).

2. In the collage, write or represent the different people, what you associate them with, activities shared with them. What do they give you, what do you give them? Go beyond your family to include people in the community who you might not have much direct contact with but they are part of community support.

3. How important is this relationship to you and why? Would you make an effort to maintain the friendship or let it slip away if that person didn't make any effort toward you?

4. If you had a problem, who would you ask to help? Have you done that before? What was the outcome?

5. Have you helped people in the collage? Did they ask for your help or was it unspoken? How did it feel to help someone else?

6. Would you like to make any of these connections stronger? If you wanted to make any particular relationship stronger, what actions could you take? Focus on positive relationships as a resource for resilience.

7. Finally, sometimes we meet someone just once or know them only briefly but they have a great impact on our lives. It may have been just

one sentence from a stranger, or unexpected help from someone you hardly knew. Has anyone made a positive impression on your life in that way? If so, how? What are some things that can be said or done that can cost other people little time or effort but have tremendous positive influence? What can we do for other people to have a positive effect in similar ways?

## Connectedness

The following themes can be explored with expressive art and/or mind maps:

- Family.
- Sharing.
- This group.
- Being this age.
- What do you like about your family? What don't you like?
- What do you like best about your closest friend?
- What makes you a good friend?
- How do you think other people see you?
- What do you find interesting about other people?
- What are things that you think are interesting about you and may be good topics of conversation?

Choose a theme or no theme – do a group art work, sharing paint and paper, working in and around each other.

### Working relationships

For many people with Asperger's Syndrome, work is very important. If they are working in an area that they enjoy, it can become the most important aspect of their lives. In a working environment, however, relationships can have hidden agendas that the AS individual is not aware of. Similarly, there are some relationships in college where competitiveness or opposition can be hurtful.

The AS individual is generally open handed and open hearted. It is a puzzle to him or her when that generosity is misunderstood or used against them. Fortunately, there are usually some genuine and nurturing people as well. Discerning who the nurturers are and who the "predators" are will be a lifelong process. Parents can help students to identify those who are genuine and those who are not. A key is to look for patterns in behavior – an AS trait is to take words literally and inconsistencies between words and actions should be recognized. The same principles are likely to apply in more mature relationships:

- Is a new friend consistent or do they "blow hot and cold"?
- Do they need your help but rarely give back?
- Do they speak negatively about other people and past friends?
- Is there someone you trust who can give a "second opinion"?

Discuss in a group real-life situations of friendships that have failed, people who have disappointed, and lessons that have been learned in those experiences. What are red warning flags that a person may not be the friend that they claim to be? What are red warning flags that even though you are putting effort into a friendship, your friendship is not wanted?

Nobody is perfect, just as we are not perfect. Flexibility and forgiveness are essential in friendship and working relationships. But at what point do we draw the line and decide that the friendship is not wanted by the other person as much as you want it, or that the other person is not genuine? What are appropriate ways of withdrawing from a friendship?

## 7.2 Concept of loyalty

Discussion, creative writing.

### Objective

Understand the concept of loyalty.

### Implementation

1. Discuss: What is loyalty? What are examples of it? How have you experienced loyalty? How have you given loyalty?

2. Write a narrative, a story, or a script for puppets/drama. In it, tell a story of loyalty, true or fiction.

3. Your friend Ben can be a bit silly sometimes. One day, while the teacher is writing on the board, he uses a slingshot to shoot a small stone in her direction and it hits her on the head. The teacher is furious. She demands

to know who hit her with the stone. She's so mad she says the whole class will stay in their seats until she finds out who hit her.

- What will you do?
- What are the reasons for doing what you do?
- In other situations, what makes the difference between when you are loyal to a friend and when you might decide that loyalty isn't appropriate? Give specific examples.
- Depending on the maturity of the group, the group facilitator may introduce real-life situations such as abuse of prison inmates and real-life dilemmas relating to divided loyalties.

## 7.3 Levels of friendship

Discussion.

### Objective

Identify different levels of friendship and appropriate behaviors.

### Implementation

Discuss and compare different real-life relationships and rate them according to the following labels:

- affection
- reciprocity of support
- love
- acquaintance
- best friend
- friends
- boyfriend/girlfriend
- intimacy
- close family, distant family.

1. What are the things that differentiate an acquaintance from a friend? The behaviors in the list above describe the differences in relationships (you may be affectionate toward distant family but love a best friend). What behaviors are appropriate to some of the relationships in the list above but not to others? What might people expect from us in different relationships? Should you send birthday cards to everyone? Invite

everyone to your wedding? Is it appropriate to talk to all of these people about a problem you are having with your boyfriend or girlfriend?

2.  How do you identify when physically close behavior is inappropriate for the level of friendship? (For example, when is a close hug acceptable and when isn't it?) What are appropriate ways of moving away from someone who is too physical for your comfort?

## 7.4 Masks of each other

Mixed media.

### Objective

Identify how other people see us.

### Implementation

1.  In pairs, each person makes a mask or painting of their partner. They may add symbols, words or colors. How do they see that person? What assumptions are made? Why? (Encourage discussion and self-revelation.)

2.  This activity has the potential to realize the impression we make on other people and with that information consider whether it is an impression we wish to make. If not, what has to be done to change it?

3.  What impression would we like to make? What would be needed to do that?

## 7.5 First impressions

Role play.

### Objective

Be self-conscious about impressions.

### Implementation

1.  You might be the smartest person in your class and be a great friend but people meeting you for the first time won't know that until they get to know you. Whether they want to get to know you (or employ you) will

depend a great deal on their first impression and the way you present yourself such as manners and dress.

2. What do people see when they first meet you? Being fashionable isn't as important as being neat and clean. The fact that everyone is unique is a wonderful thing but there are some social rules that dictate we shouldn't look too different from other people at first – we might scare them off. Ask the advice of a friend or parent about the type of clothes suitable for different situations. Find out what colors look good on you (again, ask the opinion of someone you trust).

3. Before leaving the house, stand in front of the mirror for half a minute and check – hair combed (not just the front), clean clothes, clean teeth, deodorant.

## 7.6 Appropriate conversation topics and social manners

Role play, video, improvisation, puppets.

### Objective

Practice social conversation and manners.

### Implementation

Successful social interactions require cooperative dialogue between two people – active listening skills are as important as speaking skills.

1. Initiate a conversation with another person. Possible scenes are:
   - waiting for a soccer match to start
   - a new person at school
   - another guest at a party or family wedding
   - someone older than you
   - someone the same age as you
   - a gatecrasher at your party.

2. In the role play/script, your conversation partner tells you something about themselves or that they find interesting. Ask three questions that demonstrate you have been listening, you are interested, and you would like to know more. Other ways of indicating your interest are gestures such as nodding your head, keeping eye contact. Some people lean their head slightly forward to listen – but how close is too close? Videotape

and critique later. Do you look interested even with the sound turned down?

3.  When meeting somebody for the first time, hold eye contact for at least five seconds. Shake hands, maintain about an arm's length of space between you and the other person. Be pleasant, thank people when appropriate, and say "You're welcome" when you are thanked. Sometimes it's appropriate to make "small talk." For example, you're at a party and have been left to speak with someone you've just been introduced to. Role play for two people. What are appropriate subjects? When does it become inappropriate?

4.  Role play: Someone has told you something that you don't understand. Either they spoke too quietly or quickly or used words that you didn't understand. What would be the best-mannered action? People know you are listening to them and interested in what they are saying if you ask a relevant question or say something like "That's interesting." Summarize what the person is telling you and paraphrase it in some way. If you make a habit of listening to other people, they are more likely to want to listen to you.

5.  You need to interrupt a conversation your teacher is having with someone else. What sort of things should you interrupt for? What sort of things can wait? What's the difference? Practice polite ways of interrupting someone else's conversation.

6.  What are signs that the other person might be bored? What do you do if you are bored? What are appropriate ways of finishing a conversation politely? How can you finish a conversation in a way that leaves "a link" to a possible conversation in the future?

7.  There is always the possibility that there will be people who are interested in the same things as you. This is wonderful – as long as you remember to keep a conversation open to change, allow the other person to contribute or change the topic of the conversation, or even leave it if they appear ready to do so. Remember that social conversation is like tennis – catch and return the other person's ball. A one-man tennis match can't last long. Role play changing topic. In a conversation of five minutes with another person, try to smoothly introduce two new topics (a total of three topics in the five-minute conversation). One way of doing that is to pick up on something the other person has said and ask a question about it.

8.  If you feel uncomfortable speaking in a social situation, it may work to your advantage to widen your interests and be prepared to talk about a variety of things, just for the sake of social grace. What are appropriate social conversation topics? Discuss some appropriate topics, keeping in

mind that very personal information and questions sometimes make other people uncomfortable.

9. What are social manners? One definition of manners is the skill of making other people comfortable. Discuss the items in the list below and where they are on the 1–10 Good Manners Scale (a scale invented just for this exercise). Explain why you gave them the manners score that you did:

   - approaching a person who is alone at school and initiating a conversation with them
   - asking someone how much they earn
   - wanting to leave a conversation with someone and telling them "Gotta go" and going
   - leaving a conversation with "It was very pleasant speaking to you but I'd rather speak to Tom"
   - leaving a conversation with "I have to go to the bathroom now"
   - finishing a conversation with someone in a party – and leaving them to stand in the middle of the room on their own
   - finishing a conversation with "I've really enjoyed speaking with you but I have to go now. I hope we can speak again next time"
   - speaking with your mouth full of food.

10. With a book of social etiquette suitable for the age group, culture, and situations that group members are likely to encounter, use drama and role play to enact and practice social manners. There are also good videos available on this subject. Watch as a group and discuss, generalizing to real-life situations and role playing.

## 7.7 Conversation: reacting appropriately

Role play, video, improvisation, puppetry.

### Objective

Practice appropriate responses to other people.

### Implementation

1. You are at a party and someone you've never met begins an argument with you. Perhaps they've had too much to drink but they are very aggressive. What is the appropriate response?

2.    Someone at school or college begins rumors about you – tells a teacher that you have cheated. What is the appropriate response?

3.    You've started to drive and a policeman pulls you up and tells you that you were driving dangerously. You don't think you were. What is the appropriate response? Can you think of other scenarios where you might be tempted to act without thinking about all the possible consequences?

4.    Other themes to practice conversation (beginning, responding, finishing):

- It's your first day at a school and you are lost – ask someone for help and introduce yourself at the same time.

- It is lunchtime at school – ask someone if you can sit with them and have a short conversation with them.

- There is a new person at school – introduce yourself and welcome them, finish the conversation by suggesting seeing them again in the future.

- You would like to share a school project with someone – approach someone and have a discussion about it.

- Your new friend wants you to cut school and go to the mall. How might the discussion go?

- You are eating lunch with a friend called Chris. Thomas, who is mean to Chris, approaches you and wants you to leave your friend Chris and look at his new computer game. What would you say?

- You don't understand the way the teacher explained a math problem at school. You have asked him to tell you again but he got angry, saying you weren't concentrating. What could you say?

- Have a conversation with someone that goes for five minutes and in that conversation find out five things about them, including how they like their school, and finishing by suggesting that you meet later.

- You are having a conversation with your friend Chris but all he wants to talk about today is his new dog. He's very excited about it. How might that conversation go?

- Your friend John likes a girl called Kate and talks about her all the time. You don't see what all the fuss is about and would prefer to talk about something you are interested in. How would you deal with that?

- A friend tells you he can get some drugs if you want some. How might that conversation go?

- Someone at school laughs at the clothes you wear. That hurts your feelings but you want to be friends.

- You are talking in a group of five people and disagree with all of them on what movie you should go and see. What is an appropriate conversation?

- You are speaking with a friend who changes topic in the conversation very often. In this conversation, he talks about his dog, his homework, a plane in the sky, what he wants for Christmas, and how hungry he is. What can you contribute to the conversation?

- Chris's new dog ran onto the road and was hurt by a car. He is very upset and starts to cry. What conversation might you have about it?

- You will be going to college next year and you are worried about it. You have a conversation with your teacher about it and you have a conversation about your friend who is also worried about going to college. What sort of thing would you discuss with each of them?

- As well as going to college next year, what other experiences do you think you could share with your friend? Have a discussion with him about the things you are both experiencing at the moment.

## Videotaping

Videotaping interactions is a valuable tool. For individuals with Asperger's Syndrome, there may be an inconsistency between how they see themselves (and their behavior) and what is apparent to other people. Because of this there are often misunderstandings with other people and hiccups in social interaction. Videotaping allows the actor to see what other people see, assess the appropriateness and effect of subtle behaviors, and modify them if appropriate. Videotaping allows a realistic check on modifications to behavior.

## 7.8 Open-ended questions, extending conversation

Role play, puppetry, videotaping.

To build friendships and relationships, we need to be interested in other people. We need to show them we are interested in the conversation by listening to them and talking about what is interesting to them. Very often a person with AS unintentionally leads or dominates a conversation according to their agenda. This activity introduces a couple of strategies that extend a conversation, show interest in other people, and let other people talk about themselves rather than one person dominating the conversation.

## Objective

Use open-ended questions to extend a conversation. Practice listening skills.

## Implementation

1.  Form groups of three people. It is the role of one person to question the other two. The first person is interested in doing a science class that the other two have already done. He is also interested in being friendly and extending a conversation with both of them.

2.  To gain more information about the science course he would like to do, he asks one person a "close-ended question": "Did you like the science class with Mr. Bratt?" He then asks the third person of the group an open-ended question: "What did you think about the science class with Mr. Bratt?" Let the conversation extend as long as feels comfortable for all participants. Videotape the conversation and critique it later. Which type of questions result in the best answers? Identify the difference between a closed and open questioning style and what each contributes to the conversation.

3.  For the sake of being friendly and extending a conversation, the first person asks one of the others, "Do you want to go to the mall?" He then says to the third person in the group, "I hear there's a sale of video games on at the mall and I was thinking of going up to have a look. What video games do you like?" Encourage the third person to talk about themselves and what they like. Let the conversation extend as long as feels comfortable.

4.  Look at the videotape of the conversations and make note of which question/statement elicited most information and which question opened the door toward building a friendship.

     Typically, a close-ended question gets a one or two word answer. Someone has asked for a fact, a concrete response, leaving little room for ongoing conversation.

     An open-ended question asks for more information and the nature of the question requires more of a contribution from the other person.

     Sometimes a conversation can be extended simply by making an observation. "You look tired" or "You're angry" invites the other person to comment. A simple word like "Wow" tells the person you are listening to what he has to say and encourages him to continue.

5.  Listen carefully to what the other person is saying. Pick up a piece of it and ask a question about it to develop the conversation further. For example, if the first person says "I preferred art to science," the listener can show interest and extend the conversation by saying "What sort of things did you do in art?"

6.  Practice open-ended questions and statements. Practice listening and asking questions related to new information that is brought into the conversation. The goal is to encourage the other person to talk and keep the conversation going. Below are some suggested themes:

    - You and Ben had an argument and you want to find out whether Ben is still mad at you.

    - You saw Joe at the soccer match with a new guy and you want to find out who it was.

    - You would like to go to soccer with your friends on the weekend and don't know if Mum will let you.

    - You would like to initiate a conversation with someone you don't know.

## Listening

Sometimes activities finish sooner than the time allotted for them. Use these opportunities to ask members to reflect on what other members have said – or allow time specifically for these questions:

- Have they understood the essence of the other person's contribution?

- Do they understand their feelings?

- What do they have to contribute to that information?

- How do they relate – or not – to that person?

## Rhythmic matching, social synchrony

A lack of empathy is one of the most common traits of Asperger's Syndrome. "Empathy" may be the wrong word. Lack of empathy suggests a lack of warmth or compassion toward other people. In fact, AS people can be extremely warm, sincere, and friendly. A lack of "synchrony" may be a more accurate term. This is what Dr. Benjamin Boone, musician, composer, and educator, has written:

> When people speak, they choose not only the syntax, but also the rhythm, articulation, dynamic and pitch of each utterance. In this manner, all speakers instantaneously compose melodies with their voices... It is well documented that when conversing, people tend to

synchronize their body movements and speech rhythms with those of their conversation partner. For example, body movements of the listener, such as eye blinks and hand gestures, regularly occur in synchronization with the speaker's speech rhythms and/or body movements. As the intimacy level increases, so does the level of rhythmic synchrony. Such coordination conveys mutual cooperation and unites members of a group.

Such synchronization of speech and body movements between conversation partners has been shown to be so pervasive that during the playback of a recording of a typical family dinner, a coordinated ballet can be witnessed.

The following is a quote from Douglis (1987):

> You can stomp your foot to the family dinner as you could to the strains of bebop or Beethoven, once you learn to see and hear this unintentional rhythm. When family members talk, stressed syllables – emphasized by louder volume and/or change in pitch – usually carry the rhythm. Even when the conversation lapses, the beat goes on. Diners dab their napkins to the beat. Hands reach for the salt on the beat. A knife hits the plate on the beat. And when the mother gets up, her footsteps continue to tap out the pulse as clearly as a metronome would. When two conversations develop at the table…they share the same pulse.

Rhythmic matching, also known as "rhythmic synchrony," seems to be the fundamental glue by which cohesive discourse is maintained. (Boone 1989, pp.1–4)

Thus, perceived lack of empathy might be more correctly described as marching to the beat of their own drum. If, as Dr. Boone suggests, rhythmic synchrony is the fundamental glue by which cohesive conversation is maintained, activities to promote synchrony may introduce ways to put people on the same wavelength and "in tune" with each other.

The impact of lack of synchrony for people with Asperger's Syndrome is an area that is just beginning to be explored. Dr. Boone is more specific about the role that verbal and nonverbal language plays in adding to a sense of unity in social interaction.

> Research shows that synchronizing the rhythm of body movements (eye blinks, chewing, hand movement, etc.) and speech (mostly the pulse or beat which governs the more rapid surface rhythm of the speech or the body movements) is one of many ways that humans create a sense of group membership. When we want to be accepted by a group, we adopt several aspects of that group as a nonverbal way of indicating you have

something in common with them – syntax, slowing down speech, inflection – all on the subconscious level.

Additionally, conversations have rhythmic give and take. We nonverbally communicate when we have finished speaking (through rhythm, pitch, etc.), so that the other person can then speak. We are in turn quiet until they are finished. A central "beat" tends to govern such alterations in speakers. From this, we can glean that a speaker who synchronizes the rhythm of their speech with the person with whom they are speaking is sending a message akin to "I have heard you, I'm accommodating you, I am showing you I have heard you and that I am moving to accommodate you, I want to have a conversation with you, and continue the conversation, etc."

Conversely then, if someone speaks in a manner outside of the group norm, the paralinguistic message is quite different. An individual with flat, emotionless or stilted speech, who interrupts or is out of sync is viewed as not polite – he or she either does not want to be a member of the group or they are an outsider, adversely affecting interactions. (Boone 1989)

Earlier in the book, activities have been suggested to strengthen coordination of motor coordination with rhythm, including use of a metronome. They can be modified (e.g. quiet background metronome) or the following activities can be used to enhance social synchrony.

## 7.9 Rhythmic synchrony and connectedness

Poetry, music, movement.

### Objective

To listen to others and be "in tune with them."

### Implementation

1. Two people read a piece of poetry together. Try to match tone, inflection, pitch, and rhythm. Speak as one. If there is difficulty in keeping the rhythm, play a soft beat on a percussion instrument – not so loud that it leads, but softly in the background like a heartbeat to support the flow of the voices by emphasizing pattern. The goal is to reach a stage where there is a flow with both people being "in tune" with each other, synchronized in rhythm.

2. Using the same piece of poetry, and the background percussion if necessary, read alternate lines individually with a rhythmic flow in the transition. After a rhythm has been established take away the percussion.

The goal is now to be in tune with each other in a way that requires each individual to *listen*, and to synchronize to their partner's rhythm. The final goal would be to repeat this exercise with a non-rhyming piece of prose, being even more sensitive to each other and focusing on matching pitch, tone, and inflection.

3.    Integrate movement with a variation of items one and two. The two individuals do not touch but are aware of each other's bodies sharing and moving in the same space. Flow with the percussion instrument (or music), mirroring, coordinating, and matching movements (hands, arms, neck, feet, twists, turns), mood, and flow. The goal is to lose the sense of independence and become a participant, to connect and move in synchrony with music and partner.

## 7.10 Synchrony

Yoga, music, movement.

### Objective

To practice social synchrony.

### Implementation

1.    This book has recommended frequent practice of relaxation techniques. Adding a quiet background music with a soft but regular pulse may have the effect of synchronizing the mood of group members, perhaps following a similar heartbeat.

2.    Yoga or meditation are also physiologically calming and it has been found that these activities often result in common breathing patterns with other people in the room.

3.    Choreograph, rehearse, and practice interactive movement with conversation, such as clapping hands or castanets (see Metronome activities, Chapter 5).

4.    Sing in rounds, learn a simple dance with a unifying beat.

5.    Encourage group members to move in and around each other's space in time with music or percussion – a form of movement or creative dance. It may be easier to practice spatial coordination by moving together within a circle of elastic or lycra (Dunphy and Scott 2003).

## 7.11 Mirrors

Movement.

### Objective

To observe and focus on the details of another person's movements and coordinate action with them; concentration.

### Implementation

1.  Standing on either side of a line on the floor, two actors face each other, in the same posture as though looking at themselves in a mirror.

2.  The first actor makes a facial expression, or moves a limb, maintaining eye contact with the second person.

3.  The second person mimics as closely as possible the first person, being the "reflection in the mirror." After about one minute the roles are reversed and the first actor mimics the second actor. Mood music may help establish a rhythm, even if the movements aren't mirrored precisely.

## 7.12 Drumming and percussion

Percussion circle.

### Objective

Develop expression within a group.

Drum and percussion circles are ideal and engaging creative expressive activities. They lend themselves to developing rhythmic synchrony, teamwork and cooperation, individual expression within a group context, social interaction, coordination and motor skills, expression of emotion, and release of stress. A "conversation" can be developed using sound as language without the need for words. A very useful link for program information and finding local and international drummers/teachers/therapists is the website for the Rhythmic Arts Project founded by Eddie Tuduri: www.traponline.com. The site also offers information on guides to beginning a drumming program.

## Music therapy

Because Asperger's Syndrome is multifaceted and affects a range of senses, interventions ideally address and attempt to integrate the various facets and senses. Music therapy is a specialized profession that taps unconventional learning methods and combines auditory and vocal senses with social interaction. Three exercises below illustrate a few of the ways that music can be applied as a therapeutic activity.

In these exercises, singing is used to practice clear and rhythmic enunciation and articulation of words, pitch, and expression. "Chaining" is a technique of identifying steps and sequencing in the performance of a task. Learning through modeling is making connections between seeing and learning. Accompanying requires "listening" (vs. hearing which is passive) and expressing, cooperation and teamwork, social connection, and motor skills and coordination (when dance or movement are involved).

Many thanks to Jayne Standley RMT-BC, Ph.D, Professor of Music Therapy and Director of the Music Therapy Program at the Florida State University, for this contribution. She is the author of *Music Techniques in Therapy, Counseling, and Special Education* (1991), which is recommended as a versatile and practical tool for professionals, and editor of the *Journal of Music Therapy*.

## 7.13 Music therapy #1

Learning a song.

### Objective

Accompany with the most advanced technique of which you are capable on guitar, autoharp, or keyboard and teach group to sing a new song.

### Preparation

1. Select a non-religious song that is probably unknown by peers.
2. Practice and memorize accompaniment.
3. Practice giving starting pitch, singing, and accompanying each line, then chaining lines together.

### Implementation

1. Sing one verse of song with accompaniment for group.

2.  Make eye contact with all members and assess those who appear to be listening. If members appear bored, change something you are doing; for example, talk more softly, speed up pacing, move closer to group, etc.

3.  Tell group that you will sing one line while they listen and then they will sing along with you.

4.  Say "Listen" and sing the first line.

5.  Give starting pitch, cue group entry, and lead them in singing first line.

6.  Repeat steps four and five until 80 percent of group are accurate.

7.  Nonverbally encourage singing, participation, eye contact, etc.

8.  Sing first line with group, say "Listen," and continue singing second line.

9.  Say "Sing," give starting pitch and entry cue, and lead group in singing second line.

10. Repeat singing second line until 80 percent of the group are accurate. Continue scanning group to assess accuracy, enjoyment, and participation.

11. Say "Beginning," give starting pitch, first word of song, and entry cue, lead group in singing lines one and two together. Repeat until accurate.

12. Teach each subsequent line using this chaining procedure until entire song is learned. Correct any musical inaccuracies by singing correctly for group followed by their repeating your modeling.

13. Encourage participation, eye contact, enjoyment, etc. through teaching phase.

## NOTE

The objective of the above technique is to teach quickly and efficiently while maintaining a high level of group interest and musical accuracy. Little or no talking should be required and occasions of stopping the flow of music should be reduced to a minimum.

## MUSIC SPECIFICATIONS

1.  Song should be appropriate to peer level and interest but probably new to majority of group.

2.  Song should have at least two verses and chorus (or 12 lines).

3.  Use most advanced accompaniment techniques of which you are capable on guitar, autoharp, or keyboard.

## 7.14 Music therapy #2

Learning a dance.

### Objective

Teach a simple dance of at least ten different sequential steps.

### Preparation

1. Select dance steps and music, synchronize steps with music, and design cues for each step. Use chaining procedure to teach routine. (Adapt the chaining procedure used in activity 7.13.)

2. Practice and memorize dance and chaining routine.

### Implementation

1. Teach a dance using cueing, chaining, and correction. Scan group continuously to assess those who require assistance. Correct.

2. Encourage participation, enjoyment, rhythmic accuracy.

3. Ensure that the tempo of dance matches that of recording during practice.

4. Turn on music and perform dance.

MUSIC SPECIFICATIONS

Recorded song, moderate tempo, obvious beat of probable interest to peers.

## 7.15 Music therapy #3

Learning two guitar chords (see Figure 7.1).

### Objective

Use color coding system to teach two chords on the guitar.

### Preparation

1. Prepare guitar with red dots (numbered 1, 2, 3) on frets for finger placement of C chord and numbered blue dots for G7.

2. Practice teaching procedure in implementation, especially step 11.

3. Place guitars on floor in front on chairs prior to beginning.

## Implementation

1.  State task in one sentence.

2.  Instruct group to pick up guitars but not to lay them.

3.  Quickly and briefly approve specific individuals as they follow instructions.

4.  Show the group correct position of guitar on lap. Scan group, correcting any who require it.

5.  Direct group to place left hand on the three red dots by specifying each finger and numbered dot in sequence. Scan group, correcting any who require it.

6.  Direct group to press all fingers on dots and to reach right hand across and strum once across all strings, modeling these steps as you say them. Correct anyone who made an error.

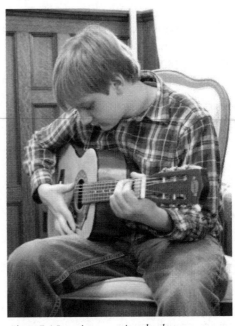

*Figure 7.1 Learning two guitar chords*

7.  Say "Listen" and demonstrate four strums on this chord in rhythm of song while nodding head in rhythm.

8.  Say "Play and strum four times on this chord in rhythm with me. Ready, begin." Use strum hand for entry cue.

9.  Praise those who are correct and who stop after four strums, etc. Repeat if there were errors.

10. Repeat Steps 5, 6, 7, 8, and 9 for blue dots.

11. Say "This time we will strum four times on red, then four times on blue. I will cue you when to change fingers. Press red and strum four times in rhythm with me. Ready, begin." Use head and strum arm for entry cue. As group begins strum four, say "Change to blue dots" and use head and arm as cue to maintain the rhythm of the next four strums. Praise those who are correct. Repeat and correct if there were errors. Encourage those who are trying, watching, listening, following directions, making music, etc.

The technique described above is a systematic task analysis of how to teach someone to lay the guitar using a color-coded system. Other chords could potentially be taught.

HINT

If there are not enough guitars for each person in the group to have one, have those persons without a guitar simulate one by practicing same procedures on their lap. Transfer guitars after Steps 9 and 10. Persons without guitars always continue to practice each step in simulation.

MUSIC SPECIFICATIONS

C and G7 chords.

## 7.16 Rhythm in a team

Group art, music, movement, synchrony.

### Objective

Identify benefits of teamwork and cooperation. Relevant to the skill level of the group, a real project might be planned and executed, such as raising money for a local community group.

### Implementation

With your group, do a synchronized activity (no, not swimming). Do a group painting/collage on a single large piece of paper, move together in each other's space to music, drum together to a piece of recorded music, each with an individual contribution but following the group rhythm and mood.

1.  What feelings do you have working in close proximity together on the same piece of paper? Happy? Awkward? Embarrassed? Do you feel you have to move out of the way of other people or are they in your way?

2.  What feelings do you have when you are "in tune" and working together harmoniously with other people on the paper? When do you experience those feelings outside the group?

A variation on the cooperative and "group art" theme is for the group to take each other's hands and feet and take artistic license with them, applying paint on the paper.

## 7.17 Teamwork

Collage, team mind map.

### Objective

Identify benefits of teamwork and cooperation.

### Implementation

ACTIVITY #1

As a group, do a *team* mind map/collage with "teamwork/cooperation" as the theme:

- What are the advantages and disadvantages of working with a team?
- When has working as a team not worked out for you? Why didn't it work?
- What are personal characteristics that can damage cooperative relationships? For example, explore the possible repercussions if one person makes most of the decisions and is dominating.
- What are personal characteristics that help a team work together successfully? For example, think of real-life situations that you have experienced where everyone worked together well. Who were the influential members of that group and what did they contribute?
- What personal characteristics do you have that would make a contribution to a cooperative team?

ACTIVITY #2

Role play the following situation and improvise potential outcomes.

A teacher has asked a small group of students to make a project of working together as a team. The goal is to raise as much money as possible for the local animal shelter in a month. Tom immediately tells everyone how he should be the team leader because he loves dogs, has always owned dogs, and had a dog that won a ribbon at a dog show. His team members are nice to him and say, "That's nice but this is not about prize dogs – it's about raising money for homeless dogs." Tom immediately tells everyone how good he is at that too. He has raised money for charities before – he even won an award for it and met the mayor who told him he was fantastic and he got his picture in the paper for all the money he'd raised and then the local television news interviewed him and in fact he could call the television reporter right now and get him to do a story on raising money for this project.

Tom is indeed good at what he does and clever and might make a good team leader, but everything he says makes his team members mad. Why? Would they want him as their team leader? Why not? What are words for this sort of verbal behavior?

Even if Tom had the wonderful skills he told everybody about (which I'm sure he has because AS individuals are typically so honest), what would have been more positive ways of using those skills in a team? What were more positive ways he could have offered to help? If you were in Tom's team, what could you say to him to show him the error of his ways in a friendly and diplomatic way?

## 7.18 Newsletter

Group activity, writing.

### Objective

Practice teamwork. Build connections, a network of people with similar interests.

### Implementation

Form a casual "club" with group members. If groups are facilitated in a larger facility such as a health clinic or support center, make connections with other groups. Write a newsletter with news, personal stories, and successes of club members, photos of their art works, and advising of upcoming social events such as group trips to a restaurant, theater, or fun park. As a club, contact similar AS support groups and arrange trips together.

## Problem solving in a team

Problem solving often requires cooperation with other people. In a team, it also requires language and listening skills. Even if the problem is personal, discussing it with trusted others is helpful. With help, larger problems can be broken down into smaller manageable pieces, different perspectives considered, possible solutions explored, and feasible goals determined. The purposeful behavior in problem solving also requires attention and the ability to concentrate. Social and emotional skills play a central role in how a problem is defined and managed.

### Some strategies for problem solving in a team

1.  *Verbal brainstorming*: discussion/description/alternate perceptions and projected outcomes.

2. *Visual association techniques*: spider mind, mind mapping, flow charts.

3. *Different perceptions*: other people's experience or structured through a Thinking Cap type exercise (green = positive; yellow = alternative, etc.).

4. *Cause and effect diagrams.*

5. *ABC technique.*

## 7.19 ABC problem solving in a team

Cognitive behavioral.

### Objective

In a team, apply ABC technique to problems. Solving a dilemma is not as important in this activity as learning to work in a team, being willing to listen to other people's point of view, acknowledging other feelings and perspectives, contributing suggestions without being controlling, accepting suggestions as valid even if there is disagreement, building an environment of personal support. Support this activity with a visual reminder of the three steps for reinforcement.

> **A** *Adversity* or *Antecedent* (problem, difficult situation or relationship)
>
> **B** *Beliefs* and thoughts about the adversity/situation/relationship that is causing stress
>
> **C** *Consequences* (thoughts and behaviors).

Point out the common tendency to experience "thinking traps" (Reivich and Shatte 2002) and the need to be aware of them to question the validity of beliefs. Ask group members to make note of those thinking traps that they may commonly fall into.

### Implementation

#### A = ADVERSITY OR ANTECEDENT

What is a real-life problem for you? Perhaps your parents don't want you to drive, or you're anxious about traveling on your own, or you don't want to come to these groups. Identify the problem and write it down. Discuss it with group members. They may have a similar experience or they may have valuable information to offer because they are not emotionally biased or have a different perspective. Examples:

- All of your friends not only drive, but most of them have cars – you're dependent on them.

- You have to travel to England and it will require you to take public transport, catch buses and planes on your own, and carry a number of bags.

- You don't like coming to these groups – they're a waste of your time, you don't like the leader, you'd rather watch television at home.

### B = BELIEFS AND THOUGHTS #1

Write a list of associated thoughts and beliefs. Explore all associations. Perhaps drawing images will help you. What do you think of when you think about the problem? What are you feeling? You don't have to have reasons for your feelings – just write them down.

- You feel embarrassed because you have to ask friends to give you a lift, you are angry because your parents don't trust you, they never let you do anything on your own, they'll keep you home forever if they can.

- Traveling to England will be scary, you won't be able to understand the currency or rules; it will be hard to carry all the bags and you'll probably get lost.

- Coming to these groups makes you feel like there's something wrong with you – you lie to your friends about where you go in case they tease you. It's boring and nobody likes you.

### B = BELIEFS AND THOUGHTS #2

Now use the team to question your thoughts and beliefs. Nobody can question how you feel about a situation, but they can question the validity or truth of your feelings. If you're embarrassed, why are you embarrassed? Do you think you're not as good as other people? Question that thought. How do you know you're not as good as other people?

Use the team to ask them what their perspective is on your beliefs. Perhaps they think you are over-reacting. Are you prepared to listen to their point of view? Go through the list of thoughts and beliefs and question every one of them. Think about possible alternative thoughts. Where is the evidence that the reality matches your thoughts and beliefs?

Beside every thought and belief from the previous list, with group members, think of a few alternative possibilities and pick one – the most likely.

C = CONSEQUENCES

Work through the list. Often other people see the same situations differently. If it's possible that other perspectives are true, what would the consequences be?

If there is a possibility that people don't like you because they don't know you, perhaps you could be more open to them. They could get to know you and you could make new friends.

Discuss in the group the following common reasons for faulty beliefs. Be open to each other's constructive criticism. Practice making constructive criticism kindly. Common reasons for faulty beliefs include:

- jumping to conclusions
- tunnel vision
- magnifying and minimizing
- personalizing
- externalizing
- overgeneralizing
- mind reading or believing we know what other people are thinking
- emotional reasoning – drawing assumptions based on emotion.

# 7.20 The island

Group activity, paper mâché, mixed media.

## Objective

To be playful and have fun (important for a positive life), use imagination, organization skills, cooperation, and teamwork. This activity can be tailored to the skill and interest levels of participants. There is scope to make it sophisticated and introduce conceptual themes for discussion (what social services should we provide?) or can be kept to a simple group sculpture activity. At any level, strategies for working as a cooperative team should be emphasized.

## Implementation

1. With team members, brainstorm ideas for an island that you can design to be perfect. What would it look like? What would some of the elements be? What would the temperature and weather be? What sort of water is around the island, what sort of geography does the island have?

2.  With a large piece of paper in the middle of the table and group members seated more or less evenly around it, each person draws the coastline of his section of the island, considering the elements just discussed.

3.  Appoint a government, a governor, people in office with different responsibilities, democratic "rules" for voting on decisions. Using democracy, design a flag for the island, name the island.

4.  Socially, would there be a place for privacy and public life? Would everyone live together or in separate places? What about leisure activities? Keeping in mind the geography of the island, allocate different areas for different functions.

5.  What would be the budgeting priorities of the local government? What will the main income of the island be? How can that be used to the advantage of most people on the island without disadvantaging others?

6.  If there are problems that affect the community, how should they be solved? (Someone on the island is behaving very badly – what should be done with him?)

## Reading social cues and social interaction

Social skill development is an important part of support for the adolescent with AS traits. At home, living by their own rules, there is limited social interaction. Work environments cause stress but social interaction is usually structured, limited, and predictable. It is in the social world of meeting new people, friendships, dating, leisure and community activities that the individual may be at a loss, not knowing what to say, and being misunderstood by other people.

It is those who go out and interact, take risks, and learn through experience who will become more adept at social interaction while those who are comfortable at home are less likely to develop appropriate life skills. Support for the adolescent involves thinking about, discussing, role playing, and practicing social interaction in as many forms as possible. Having genuine and generous friendships offers informal learning through example and modeling.

Some individuals may need to learn concrete phrases to keep a conversation going. All will become more skilled at interacting in novel social situations through practice of listening and speaking skills, understanding expectations, seeing another person's perspective, and learning to detect and decode social cues.

For younger children, an effective learning strategy has been developed by Carol Gray (1994). Children develop a language of symbols which can be used as a sort of shorthand in cartoons. Emotion and other unspoken factors which play into conversation are represented in the cartoons by balloons, thought clouds, colors, and shapes.

Social stories can be more sophisticated for older individuals. Drama, role plays, and puppetry provide opportunities to act out previously scripted or cartooned social themes and stories. Drama is the ideal creative activity to learn face and body cues, match them to mood and intention, practice conversation, detect clues in a conversation partner's gestures or voice, and deal with hypothetical situations through conversation. Activities related to drama stimulate imagination and creativity and offer opportunities for social interaction where alternatives in reactions and outcomes can be explored and practiced.

Visual supports can add humor as part of a pantomime – someone in the background waving colored paddles or balloons on cardstock with sticks, such as green for friendly, amber for be careful with your words, caution with this person, red for decidedly unfriendly, black for verbal attack, purple for flirtatiousness (a come-on) – colors to suit the theme.

Use of lights, masks, and music can also signal underlying meanings, moods, and intentions.

Themes to explore social cues and interaction can include the following:

1. Becoming friendly with a person and possibly asking them for a date.

2. Confusion and misunderstanding in conversation:

   - Sean says "Can you help me with my homework?" but David hears "Can you do my homework for me?"

   - Sean is enthusiastically talking about a movie with great special effects and David thinks he's talking about what happened over the weekend.

   - Misinterpreting the intention one person has toward another of the opposite sex.

3. Seeing somebody in pain – in the classroom, a stranger on the street, at a football game.

4. Hurt feelings – one person inadvertently not being invited to join a group of friends; a friend is hurt when his job application is rejected.

5. Annoyance – friend is tired of being interrupted all the time but is being polite about it; father is annoyed because he can't find the tool he left on the kitchen table this morning.

6. Fear – while hiking, one friend becomes frightened of the height but wants to keep going so the whole team doesn't have to turn back; a person is frightened of his friend's pet snake.

7. Boredom – one person is talking very enthusiastically about the movie he just saw but his friend is bored; three friends are sitting on the sofa watching the television together – one thinks it is wonderfully sentimental when the actor kisses the actress, another thinks kissing scenes are stupid and embarrassing; the other friend is just bored.

Embarrassment, disappointment, excitement, anticipation, sadness, impatience, concern, guilt, and suspicion are other emotions that can be detected through body language and facial cues, and acted out through improvisation or a script.

## 7.21 Movement

Group activity, music, movement.

### Objective

Use music to express and identify social cues and emotions.

### Implementation

1. Choose two different types of music – one sad and tragic, the other uplifting. Ask group members to move their bodies and faces according to how the music makes them feel. If convenient, take photographs or video for an external perspective. Afterward, discuss how music can change mood. The same group, in the same room, in the same circumstances, will probably have felt different things. How are those things represented visually in the photographs or video?

2. Watch a music video and discuss the impression that it gives and the feelings it invokes. Discriminate between tone, loudness, clothes, words, music itself, color, speed, light. What do they each contribute to the overall impression?

3. Draw a cartoon mockup of a music video that group members might produce for a particular song. Pay attention to the visual details and what they contribute to the overall image and character of the video. Ask group members to work as a team and justify why different details were used and what effect they were expected to contribute to the overall impression.

### Storytelling and scriptwriting

Storytelling and scriptwriting are therapeutic in themselves when used to express perspectives and feelings. They also offer opportunities to express the perspectives and feelings of other people. Storytelling and scriptwriting offer the opportunity to elaborate on interaction and/or details that the storyteller feels are important but may otherwise go unnoticed. As a link between a story and its drama, a script details verbal and physical social behaviors, encouraging awareness of both. In all cases, being able to tell a story in a way that engages other people is a skill to be practiced and developed.

## 7.22 Reading social cues #1

Storytelling, scriptwriting.

### Objective

Use sequencing, improvisation, and imagination, possibly different perspectives, in retelling a coherent story.

### Implementation

1. The group leader tells a basic story (designed to suit skill level) with a theme that involves social interaction and behavior, such as the following:

   • family dinner

   • friendships

   • making a new friend

   • an embarrassing situation.

2. Group participants identify basic elements of the story – who said what; what was the reaction and repercussions of someone's words or behavior. Make note of social behavior – the story that is told through actions not words. For example, Johnny may compliment his aunt on the dinner, then quietly slip it to the dog under the table.

3. Participants may do a cartoon (script) of the basic story to provide a visual representation of the basic elements. The cartoon indicates who is involved, the actions, context. Headings or voice balloons can be used to indicate changes in direction and speech.

4. Using the same basic elements, take turns in elaborating and improvising on the story with variations. Keep to the main storyline but tell it in a different way – possibly from someone else's perspective or from a different time or place. In the initial instructions, tell participants that they will be randomly chosen to repeat someone's story. Attentive listening is important.

5. Points to remember are:

   • cohesiveness – don't stray too far from the main story line and bore listeners or go off on tangents

   • make clear and well-constructed sentences – picture them in your head first if necessary

   • be consistent with words and behavior of characters/actors and to the reaction of others to their words and behavior

   • be descriptive – paint a picture for the listeners that excites them even though they've already heard this story

   • when the script is read, pronounce words clearly and use interesting and variable tone of voice.

## 7.23 Reading social cues #2

Storytelling, scriptwriting, picture interpretation.

### Objective

Use imagination to tell a story.

### Implementation

Produce a picture or poster that suggests a story and ask for an interpretation of it. For example, posters of Norman Rockwell's paintings (good size for a group and available cheaply) are very suitable because the facial expressions are exaggerated, almost caricatures, yet invoke emotions and empathy. These posters can be wonderful sources of humor, storytelling, imagination, identification, and mimicry.

## Drama as therapy

Drama has been suggested as a strategy for expression and rehearsal. Integrating drama as therapy involves direct participation and interaction of an individual through:

- acting, role playing, and improvisation
- projection through puppets, dolls, and directing others.

Drama can be:

- spontaneous and improvised
- structured and planned
- directed by the facilitator
- written by participants.

Props and associated paraphernalia play a role – scenery, costumes, masks, sound, lights that require coordination in the planning and execution. There are many opportunities for hypothetical and holistic thinking. Because many of the facets related to drama have their own contribution to make to adolescent support, they are addressed separately.

## Sensory integration

As a whole, drama-related exercises provide endless potential for sensory integration – the combination and integration of visual, auditory, tactile, and body awareness senses. Drama utilizes imagination in writing a script or improvising in acting, providing opportunities to express emotion, explore personal issues and interpersonal issues. Drama gives the mature individual the opportunity to play, experiment, make mistakes, try new things, increase complexity in a safe place, stimulate neural pathways, and learn new skills.

## 7.24 Sounds

Sensory integration.

### Objective

Identify the impact of sounds around us.

### Implementation

1. Close eyes and listen to the sounds in the room around you. Open your eyes, choose materials and colors that represent those sounds for you, and put them on paper.

2.  Remember sounds that you don't like. Express what they feel like through art materials.

3.  Listen to music and draw the shapes, lines, and colors of the sounds. Can also be a rhythmic or relaxation exercise.

## 7.25 Voice exercises

Group exercises, percussion.

### Objective

Build expressive and articulation skills.

One of the benefits of drama is the opportunity to practice articulation and voice projection. Difficulty in articulation is a common AS trait. Words might be mumbled, low, slow, and slurred; they are more often fast and furious. Flat affect, or lack of emotional expression, in language is also common. Drama requires self-regulation of speech and can set up a rhythm in the conversation between actors.

### Implementation

1.  Prepare a list of different phrases or sentences. Examples are: "I'd rather be at the shore now" or "You're looking just great today." Group members can experiment with different ways of saying each phrase, one at a time, to express different emotions, or each member can take a separate phrase and see how many different ways its meaning can be changed through expression.

2.  Rhythm can be built by reciting a poem together with percussion in the background. Mirror the rhythm (fast, slow) and mood (loud, soft) of the percussion in the way the words are expressed.

## Characterizations

Examination and discussion of character could include the following:

1.  Discussion of "character." What makes a grandpa character distinctly different to a teenage character? Are all grandpa characters the same? What could distinguish between grandpas (walk, voice, attitude, gestures, weak or strong, personality, "props" such as glasses, walking stick, newspaper)?

2. What characterizes a person who is cool, sick, crazy, angry, old, very young, weird, confident, shy?

3. How are the differences demonstrated in their walk, facial expressions, speech, clothes, or props? Do you have other ideas for characters with specific mannerisms?

4. Discuss how you might open a conversation with each of these characters, or a list of other characters. For example, what would be some things you could say to an old person to begin a conversation with them? How might you begin a conversation with a musician? Or someone with a dog?

5. With a partner, develop a character, either imagined or real, and write down five to ten things about that person that is "characteristic" of them. Improvise a skit for the rest of the group in which each person acts out the character they have developed.

6. In another improvisation, similar to the first, have the character act out something without words – a mime. Express a range of emotions. Videotape. Other group members can develop a story from interpretation of emotions from posture, gestures, facial expressions. Discuss what cues indicated emotions or suggested a storyline. Play back the videotape, have group members do "voiceovers" with their storyline, and see how well their story matches the acting.

7. Do a painting/collage that expresses the character you have developed. In the collage, pieces of the person's past can be incorporated, perhaps their work, friends and family. Are the different pieces cohesive? (If the character is a grandpa, are his grandchildren important to him? What would his home look like and why? Are these things represented in the painting/collage?)

8. How is the character different to you? Think of a fear you have – perhaps fear of going out or meeting new people. Would this character react to those things the same way you do? How would he or she be different? (Drama gives opportunities to explore alternative ways of thinking.)

# Props

The way a person is dressed or their external paraphernalia can be represented by props in drama and offer clues in understanding a perspective different to our own. The man in a wheelchair sees things differently to the athlete. The rapper sees things differently to the soccer player. We cannot generalize about people (all soccer players don't see things the same way), but the way people dress can offer clues to possible differences or similarities.

If you met someone in a wheelchair and wanted to spend more time with them, what activities would you suggest? How would that differ if you met a person dressed as a rapper, or a football player? Following the same principle, people will assume things about our character in the way we dress, whether or not we wear shoes, chew gum, carry a musical instrument, and so on.

Props could be used in a number of ways such as:

1.   Supply a large box or washing basket of props – lengths of different fabrics, props, etc. Each group member takes a piece of cloth and decorates it, drapes it, and wears it in a way that suggests a character. You may add jewelry, shoes, or pieces that are not garments but add to the character.

2.   Take a piece of plain fabric – a scarf or a sheet – and move with it in a way that suggests emotion and character, not as a garment but as an extension of self.

In *Freedom to Move* (2003), Kim Dunphy and Jenny Scott suggest props such as ribbon sticks (ribbons pinned onto the end of a wooden chopstick) and parachutes or "silky" car covers for whole group movement and sculpture. Creative movement, dance, and musical activities can be combined with story-telling, performance, and film, each of which contribute opportunities for individual expression and skill building.

## 7.26 Using props

Group activity, props.

Props such as scarves, fans, masks, cloaks, hats, clothing, walking sticks, etc. encourage imagination and can also initiate different types of movement – even improvised and creative dance.

### Objective

Use movement and props to express self and emotions.

## Implementation

1. Invite each group member to choose one or two articles from an assortment of props (fabric, hats, costume accessories). Invite each to use their fabric or props in a way that reflects the rhythm and mood of the music.

2. Using the props for clues, adopt a different persona and respond and move to the music from that perspective (glittering fabric/princess; construction hat/worker; gloves/hands). Use facial expressions to add to the depth of the activity. Group members discuss how the hats/shoes/cloaks may have provoked change in what they were feeling.

## 7.27 Masks as props

Group activity, masks.

### Objective

Use masks to express emotion. Body language.

### Implementation

1. Divide the students into groups of four or five and hand out the masks. Assign them an emotional state to portray and allow them time to talk about the images that state brings.

2. Through movement enact the emotion either suggested by the mask or contrary to the mask. Other group members guess what emotion the performers are portraying and inconsistencies, if any, between mask and body language.

3. Discuss the difference between this lesson and the previous lesson on facial expressions. Talk about the challenges they faced and times when facial expressions and body language might be contradictory in real-life situations.

## Community activities

Being involved with community activities may provide a path for integrating personal interests and the positive development that is the overall goal of support. Making connections with others and community is also congruent with the Positive Psychology concept of being actively connected to something "greater than ourselves."

Horticultural activities have many potential benefits and provide opportunities to connect with the community. Working with plants has long been recognized as an emotionally soothing and physically healing activity. One of the AS traits is difficulty in seeing long-term consequences, and "stopping and starting" with various incomplete stages of a long-term project. Gardening requires long-term planning and commitment, maintenance, flexibility, and delayed gratification. Last, but certainly far from least, gardening with teenagers may inspire a new interest – one that could lead to a hobby or career.

## 7.28 Community activities
Research, oral presentation.

### Objective
Increase awareness of local community, research, cohesive presentation.

### Implementation
1. Each individual does research on local community activities that are interesting to group members. Search local newspapers and internet sites, read noticeboards, visit recreation centers such as the YMCA, or explore volunteer opportunities.

2. Each participant presents a small lecture of about five minutes about those community resources, clubs, and opportunities. Include information about how to join, benefits of joining, cost of joining, other people who are involved, and some history and activities of the organization.

3. As a group, explore opportunities that this organization may offer to develop personal interests and goals, increase knowledge, offer work opportunities, meet people and have fun.

## 7.29 Horticultural activities

Pots, plants, teamwork.

### Objective

Practice responsibility, planning, organization toward a long-term outcome or outcomes, spatial problem solving, learning from concept through process; individual or cooperatively based activities.

### Implementation

The implementation of horticultural activities will depend a great deal on age, space and time restraints, and climate. It could be one-off individual activities or an ongoing group/community project. Therefore it is difficult to detail a specific activity or activities. However, any gardening activity is likely to benefit participants because so many dimensions reinforce the strengths that enhance satisfaction and resilience.

A very good resource for activities relevant to a variety of ages (kindergarten to adult) and conditions (greenhouse, outdoor, hydroponics) is available at the website of the National Gardening Association (www.garden.org) and the associated site for children. Local nurseries can provide specific and more reliable information on suitable plants for the available space and local conditions. The following activities can be modified according to age, resources, and convenience.

1.  Containers (gourds, pots, benches) have potential to be individualized, adding to the complexity of a gardening project. Bought flowers can be put in individualized pots.

2.  Depending on climate and conditions, group members may plant a garden in an outside corner. Form a "gardening club" where a long-term project is planned and responsibility for different tasks allocated to members. Teamwork, organization, responsibility, and continuity all come into play.

3.  Paint the plants in different stages of development. Keep a journal of development along with illustrative images (as in a collage) and comments from each group member about what they learned or enjoyed on each day that they contributed to the process. This project should take five minutes a day after the initial setting up, yet offers a continuity and sense of ownership and teamwork.

4.  Connect with the community by extending the "gardening club" activities to taking plants to people in a local nursing home or children in a

hospital, and helping maintain them there. Connections to community can make an interesting photograph and story for the local newspaper, building confidence and reinforcing a sense of belonging.

## 7.30 Appreciation

A short group exercise suitable for filling in a few minutes.

*Objective*

Increase consciousness of things to appreciate or for which to be grateful.

*Implementation*

Do a round in the group, taking turns to name things for which each individual is grateful or appreciative. Be specific. One member might say "I'm grateful for my grandfather because he takes me fishing." Another might say "I'm grateful for my grandfather because he doesn't get mad when I screw up."

# Building relationships

One of the principles of the SEL model is "reflectiveness" – a "process of discovery about emotional truths or knowledge." It's a skill that applies to being able to decode the emotions, behavior, and motivations of other people – all important in building and repairing friendship.

> **Gratitude**
> Gratitude is one of the qualities associated with resilience.

## 7.31 Building relationships #1

Discussion, card.

*Objective*

Identify reasons to be grateful; acknowledge effort of other people.

## Implementation

1. In a group discussion, discuss what gratitude is and things to be grateful for. Our parents do many things for us – is that their duty or should we be grateful? If someone does what they're expected to do for us, does that mean we shouldn't be grateful?

2. Write a list of things that you can be grateful for. Who are the people associated with those things?

3. Choose one or more of those people and create a card for them that demonstrates in words or pictures – or both – your gratitude. Write words of thanks and appreciation. Decorate it in a way that shows how much you appreciate them.

## 7.32 Building relationships #2

Cards, letters, writing, art.

### Objective

Identify and practice strategies for building and repairing friendship. Decode the emotions in relationships.

### Implementation

1. You and a friend have had an argument. You lost your temper and said hurtful things. You value the friendship and want to resolve your differences. Write a card of apology. Decorate it in a way that shows how much you care about the friendship.

2. We often take our friends and relatives for granted. It's good for our relationships to reflect on them sometimes and identify what we appreciate about people – their genuineness, their help, their kindness, their tolerance. Using a mind map, explore the feelings you have about one of the people in your life. What is it that you appreciate about them? In what ways – other than a card – can you show them how much you appreciate them?

3. Role play and improvise potential outcomes to this situation: Susan is a new person to a group where you are a member. No one likes her very much because she seems to be angry at everyone else and can be very rude.

   Discuss: Try to see Susan's perspective. How do you think she is feeling? Have you ever been in that situation? What are five possible reasons she might be angry and rude? What are ways of decoding her behavior? How can we understand what might be beneath her anger and rudeness? Because we don't want to fall into the trap of jumping to conclusions, it might be wise to talk with her before making assumptions. How would you initiate a conversation with Susan to decode her behavior?

Imagine you have decided to get to know Susan better. You learn that there are some things you like about her, some things you don't. Your relationship with her doesn't just depend on how she treats you. It also depends on how you treat her. Will you focus on the things you like or the things you don't like? Imagine you are having a conversation with Susan (after the group or sharing a snack). Within that conversation you can:

- compliment her for the things you like about her *or*
- criticize her for the things you don't like about her.

What are likely outcomes? Role play. What were the differences in Susan's behavior to you in each conversation? Why do you think Susan might react differently to compliments and criticism? What are real-life examples where you have been complimented or criticized? How did you react? Of course, we may have the option of ignoring someone – neither criticism nor compliments – but this is an exercise in building relationships.

4. If there is someone at home or school who it is easy to criticize, think of something genuinely nice to say to them and compliment them instead. What was the response? Report it back to the group.

5. Practice diplomacy: You have invited a friend to go out to a party with you. You really like your friend but when he turns up it's obvious he hasn't washed. He looks really dirty and he smells. You would be embarrassed to take him to the party and as a good friend perhaps you should tell him how his dirtiness affects the way people react to him. What is a diplomatic way of discussing this with your friend? What if he takes offense? Role play.

   - What are other examples where you wonder whether you should talk to people about something that you think they need to address?

   - Have there been times when people have taken offence at what you said? Why do you think that was?

   - Are there times when it's none of your business? When do you think they might be?

   - When do you think you should use diplomacy to tell people something that might offend them?

6.  What is the appropriate way of responding to someone else's tears?

    Scene: A friend is crying. Why is she crying? What would make her feel better? Role play. (There is one simple response always appropriate in a situation where you are uncomfortable and not sure of the best thing to do. Ask. Make the observation "You're upset" and then "What can I do?" or "Can I help you?")

7.  You would like to become friends with the new girl in the class. She's very attractive and she'd be a great girlfriend. (Reverse gender if appropriate.)

    *   Why do you think she'd be a good girlfriend? What makes a good girlfriend (or boyfriend)?

    *   What are good and well-mannered ways to build a friendship?

    *   Role play a conversation with puppets. How can you impress her? What would not impress her? What's the difference between impressing and showing off? (Role play examples.) How can you leave the conversation so that a "door is open" to talking to her again? Are compliments appropriate? Can you compliment someone too much?

    *   When you really get to know someone, how can you tell them you like them? Is it necessary to tell them? If you tell them, how often should you tell them? How do you know if they like you? How do you know if they don't like you? Is it always obvious? Are people always sincere?

    *   Use your group to role play these scenarios and discuss how other group members of the opposite sex would react to different approaches. What would please them? What might embarrass them?

8.  What would you like in a friend? Form pairs in your group and interview each other as though applying for the position of "friend." Ask questions that may not be polite in real life. Discover if there are differences in what you and your partner want in a friendship, what you expect, and what you'd give. Here are some ideas to get started:

    *   Tell me about yourself.

    *   Do you think you would be a good friend? Why?

    *   What are you looking for in a friend?

    *   What is your family like? What activities do they enjoy? Do you enjoy doing things with them?

    *   Do you have a pet?

    *   How do you like school? What do you like/don't you like?

    *   What are your hobbies?

    *   What sort of work would you like to do?

    *   What activities would you enjoy with a friend?

From this information, what have you learned are differences and similarities between you and your partner? Would you be good friends for each other? Why or why not?

If your group has a newsletter, you might like to write a small article introducing your new friend to others in the group (check with him before including personal information that he told you and might not like shared with other group members).

## 7.33 Building relationships #3
Literal meanings.

### Objective
Identify the problems of literal interpretation.

### Implementation
1.  Act out the following drama, record it on videotape, and then review it as a group. A group of people are playing a game. One accidentally knocks the game off the table and spills all the pieces.

    Player #1: I'm sick of you – you always mess up the game. I was winning and now all the pieces are all over the floor. I never want to play with you again.

    Player #2: Oh, put a bag over your head. I was winning and you *always* get angry when you're losing a game.

    Player #1: I'm angry when I play with you because you're the worst player in the world – it's a waste of my time playing with you.

    Player #2: Right, and you're the world's best player! Get lost – go and cool off. [Stomps off. Finish.]

2.  Discussion:
    *   Identify examples of exaggeration or sarcasm – non-literal language.
    *   Discuss underlying meanings and implications.
    *   Discuss different ways of handling the messed up game.
    *   What are more appropriate ways of telling someone you don't want to play with them?
    *   What are appropriate ways of telling someone you're sorry you messed up the game?

- What are appropriate things to say if you are winning a game? What are appropriate things to say if you lose a game?

- Is it a waste of time to play with someone if you don't like the game? What are different perspectives of spending an hour playing a game that you don't enjoy with a friend (compromise, negotiation)?

3. Discuss the following:

- "My friend said that our teacher is crazy." Is that a fact or is that an opinion? Should it be taken literally or not?

- "The teacher said my friend is crazy." Is that a fact or is that an opinion? (Teacher's opinion is not always right.)

- "My friend says she loves her dog." Is that a fact or is that an opinion? Should I take her literally?

- "My friend says she loves Leonardo DiCaprio." Should I take her literally?

- "My friend says animals are smarter than people." Is that a fact or is that an opinion? Is it wise to take her literally?

- "My friend says she believes animals are smarter than people." Is that a fact or is that an opinion? Should this be taken literally?

- "My mom says blue is her favorite color. She also says I look good in blue." Which is fact, which is an opinion?

## 7.34 Building relationships #4

Practice.

### Objective

Build relationships with other group members.

### Implementation

1. Support groups need not always be in a closed setting. Meet each other at a coffee shop or restaurant. Democratically choose the setting, how you will get there, with whom you will go. Go in groups of three or four.

2. After the outing, discuss the questions, each offering their perception of the same outing:

- Did you look forward to the experience?

- How did you feel during the experience?

- How do you feel now about it? Would you like to do it again?

- Did you feel left out?

- Did you make an effort to include someone who might have felt left out?

- Did the details of finding a table, order, and paying the bill present any problems?

- What roles did different people play? Did everybody participate? Was one quiet? One a leader? Did that work for your group?

3. In discussion of the outing, try to assume the same social context as was in the outing – don't "take turns" – expect each to listen to the other's experiences, respond to it, ask questions of other members, not dominate the floor. Progressive feedback should be given by the group facilitator during the discussion. ("That was thoughtful of you, John, to ask how Mary felt about that.")

## 7.35 Building relationships #5

The party: discussion, role play, video.

### Objective

Identify good manners and why they are important.

### Implementation

1. If good manners are making other people feel comfortable, what can we do to make other people feel comfortable in the following situations?

   - You are introduced to someone you don't know and are now in a conversation with them. What if they are being polite but are really not interested in the conversation? (We should allow opportunities for them to change the subject or break away from the conversation. It is bad manners to leave someone on their own in the middle of the floor. A way around this is to bring one or two other people into the conversation which will make it easier for the person you are talking to – or yourself – to break away from the conversation and not leave the other there alone and feeling deserted.)

   - Are they physically comfortable? Would they like a seat? Or a drink? What is the difference between asking "Do you want" and "Would you like"?

   - What are other examples of well-mannered conversation?

- What are the unspoken rules? What would be considered "gross" behavior? What would be considered merely impolite?
- Is it good manners to gossip or talk about other people? At what point does talking about other people become bad manners?
- How do you introduce people to each other?
- What's an appropriate way to introduce yourself?
- What do you do if there is nice food on the table but no knives, forks, or plates?
- What do you do if you take a mouthful of food and it's awful?
- What do you do if someone has had too much to drink and they start arguing with you? (Don't argue back, leave the situation as quickly as possible.)
- When is it appropriate to compliment someone and why should we? What are examples of compliments?
- What do you do if someone tells a joke and you don't get it? What do you do if you tell a joke and they don't get it? How often should you tell the same joke?
- If you really like someone of the opposite gender, what are appropriate ways of expressing interest? Is it different for boys than it is for girls?
- What are appropriate sentences to finish a conversation?

2. Improvise the above "party" – have real food and drinks, a "host," chairs, props. Half the people are known to each other, the other half are "new" people. (New people can be identified with a tie around their neck or party hat.) Videotape and review afterward. Remember:

- appropriate body space and eye contact
- topics of conversation appropriate to the type of acquaintance, appropriate volume

3. Replaying the videotape allows different perspectives – what were other people experiencing in response to your behavior? Turn the sound down and look at the body language. Was there smooth changing of topics, introduction of other people, leaving conversations?

## 7.36 Building relationships #6

Manners: role play, puppetry.

### Objective

To define manners in relevant contexts, practice.

### Implementation

1. Discussion:
   - Why are manners important? Who do they serve?
   - What are examples of manners and are some more useful and important than others?
   - What's the difference between etiquette and manners (social custom vs. consideration for other people)?

2. Role play, puppetry. Practice examples of manners in the following situations:
   - interview for job application
   - making others feel comfortable in your home
   - making others feel comfortable in a place unfamiliar to you (e.g. a party)
   - asking for something
   - building a new friendship.

3. Through a humorous puppet skit, two courses of action and outcomes could be explored simultaneously. Support with visual cues, adding humor. The stage set is an office/party/appropriate context.
   - Puppeteers take turns to enact the same script on the left and right sides of the set, using the same lead-in sentences but varying on response and outcome. For example, the script begins with "Mr. Olsen, it's good to meet you. So you're interested in this job?"
   - The puppets on the right of the stage act this out, followed by a well-mannered response, "Thank you, it's a pleasure to meet you too. Yes, the job interests me very much – it would be very interesting to work here too." (A green balloon or GO sign is waved in the background, meaning, "opening the way to getting the job").
   - The puppets on the left of the stage begin with the same introductory sentence but the reaction differs. "Well, it depends if it pays good money." (A red balloon or STOP sign is waved in the background, meaning, "not a good idea if I want this job").

- The conversation moves on, alternating from side to side with different responses to the same cues.

The "alternate responses" technique can be used with a variety of themes – from problem solving to conversations with parents and teachers. The colored thought bubbles in the background are an extension of Carol Gray's Social Stories™ – colors can be used as traffic lights to visually identify the character or appropriateness of a comment or thought.

## 7.37 Job interview

Role play, video.

### Objective

Practice job interview.

### Implementation

In activity 7.36 it was suggested that manners play a part in a job interview. This activity extends that activity to practicing a job interview in all its stages.

1.  Imagine you have an appointment for a job interview. What preparation can you do before the interview itself? Discuss. Some of the points might include research on the company: What is the nature of their work? Is it a large company or small, old or new? What is the position of the person who is interviewing you?

2.  The first impression lasts longest. Before you speak the interviewer will have formed a quick impression from the way you walk into a room, are dressed, smile, shake hands. In your initial preparations for the interview, consider what you might wear. You may ask for help from family on appropriate style of clothing (applying for a part-time job at the local animal refuge will require different dress to an interview in a city office). Whatever you wear, make sure that you are clean and neat. Don't carry too many things (and don't put them on someone's desk), don't wear all your jewelry at once, and wear shoes built for comfort not a party.

    Take copies of qualifications and letters of recommendation so that your interviewer can refer to them during the interview. You can also refer to them to support your answers to the interviewer's questions. ("Why do you think you'd be good at this job?" "In her letter of recommendation, my teacher said I was good with detail, and working with accounts would require that.")

You will probably be asked at the end of the interview if you have any questions. If you like, take in a notebook and make note of questions that might arise for you during the interview. ("You mentioned that you have ongoing training seminars – could you please tell me more about that?") Writing in your notebook gives you some "time out" from eye contact but try to maintain a steady, interested (not staring) eye contact with the person interviewing you for most of the time.

3. Before you go to the interview think about what you have to offer, your strengths and skills. Letters of recommendation from people who know you (teachers, previous employers, your minister) may be more clear about your skills and will support what you say. Being employed to do work is an exchange of services. You have something to offer, and someone is willing to pay for it. Without arrogance or boasting, be aware and able to talk about two or three strengths and skills (or personality characteristics) that are "selling points" for you. What do you have to offer?

4. If you are unfamiliar with the area, give yourself lots of time to get to the place of interview. Try to arrive about ten minutes early. Be patient while waiting and don't make any comment if the interviewer is late. Don't drink coffee or eat before or during the interview.

5. When meeting your interviewer, be friendly, smile, and let him or her lead the conversation. Answer questions with a pleasant attitude but don't stray beyond the question, don't be too detailed or personal in your answers. For example, if asked why you left our last job, it's enough to say that it was a long way from home – there is no need to say how far it was, how many buses you had to take, and how early you had to leave in winter. Don't give details on office politics, gossip, and problems with people in the last job. Don't talk negatively about yourself and your abilities.

6. Most interviewers ask similar types of questions. Be prepared to answer the following type of questions:

    • Tell me about yourself. (Relate the answer to work history and personal characteristics if they are relevant to the job you are applying for.)

    • What do you enjoy about working? (Something other than "the money.")

    • Why did you leave your last job? (The prospective employer is wondering if the reason you left your last company may lead you to be unsatisfied with this company.)

    • Why would you like to work for this company?

- What previous experience have you had that would help you in this position?

- What are your personal strengths that would make you good for this position? (A way of talking about your strengths without "showing off" is to say "I've had previous experience with computers and I think that would be useful" or "Mr. ...from my last job said he appreciated that I was very punctual and careful with detail.")

- What areas do you think may cause difficulties for you? (A trick question – you want to be honest but don't put people off. Answer a question like this with a solution. For example, "Sometimes it takes me a little while to learn new things but I'm very thorough with details" or "Sometimes people take a while to get to know me but Mr. ...from my last job said in his letter of recommendation that everybody will miss me." Don't focus on negative things about yourself – redirect a question like this to a positive outcome.)

- What are your hobbies? (Relate them to how they may be useful to the job.)

- What would you do if you were given a job and it was too difficult for you? (Be confident that you will cope. Problems can be expected to arise in learning a new job and the most sensible thing to do is "ask for help.")

- What are your goals? (Keep goals related to how this job and you could work together very well – you want to work in this area, learn more about it, and will work hard to do so. Don't say your goal is to run the company or use it as a step to another better paying position elsewhere.)

7. Buy a book or do research on the internet. What makes good job interview skills? How is a good resumé written? After preparing for an interview, practice interview skills in the context of your group, role playing with an "interviewer," desk, and "office." Videotape so that you can critique your own performance.

## Bullying and unhealthy relationships

It is often assumed that bullying happens to young children. We don't talk about bullying happening to older people. We assume they can look after themselves. But bullying can become very sophisticated as its perpetrators get older. How can bullying be identified? How can it be coped with?

## 7.38 Bullying

Discussion, role play, puppetry.

### Objective

To identify bullying situations and strategies for coping.

### Implementation

1.  What is bullying? Have you experienced it? What did it feel like? Who did the bullying? How did you cope? What was the outcome? What are different forms of bullying? As we get older, how can people bully us? How can we identify if someone is being a bully? What's the difference between unfriendliness and insensitivity in someone?

2.  As a group discuss strategies of coping with unfriendliness or bullying. What are appropriate and inappropriate responses? Consider:

    *   Bullying is not just physical, it can be verbal or a threat.

    *   Identify real-life experiences that illustrate the difference between teasing and bullying. Calling names can be bullying.

    *   It is almost impossible to deal with bullies alone. Ask for help from teachers, friends, parents, and older sisters and brothers. Write down the things that are said, when, and where.

    *   Find a buddy or group of buddies. Bullies are cowards and less likely to pick on someone who has support.

    *   Practice being assertive when someone bullies you. You have the right to say "Don't do that. If you keep doing that, I'll…"

    *   Practice telling a teacher and asking for help when bullied.

## 7.39 Hate

Discussion.

### Objective

Understand the concept of hate; generalization of hate.

### Implementation

1.  Through expressive art and/or a mind map, explore all the feelings and associated personal experiences of hate.

2.  Have you ever hated someone? Who, when, why? What were surrounding circumstances? What were associated feelings?

3.  Have you felt people hated you? Who, when, why? What were surrounding circumstances? What were associated feelings?

4.  In the above examples, did you stay with the hate or move through it? Did time or circumstances change the feelings or do the feelings remain? Do you feel hate is an emotion that gives you some control or causes you to lose some control? Who controls the hate?

5.  It's impossible to like people all the time. Some people hurt us and are not likeable. What good does hate do us? What damage does hate do us? What are responses to hateful situations that could lead to outcomes that are easier to live with than hateful emotions?

6.  Have you ever heard someone say "I hate them"? What are examples of generalized hate? (That is, not hate because of what one specific person has done but hate because of what someone from their group, culture, country has done.) Discuss.

## 7.40 Harmful relationships

Handout – follow with discussion.

### Objective

Identification of harmful relationships and coping strategies.

### Implementation

1.  Give handout to group members: ask one person to read it while the others listen.

2.  Discuss the following:
    - different types of relationships and how they can enrich or hurt us
    - what makes a relationship hurtful, destructive, harmful, dangerous
    - expectations and rights
    - when things should be private, when they shouldn't – the problem with secrets
    - who you can trust, putting a support network in place
    - personal experiences.

## 7.40 Harmful relationships
### Handout

How do you recognize when a relationship is not healthy? Bullying by a casual acquaintance is fairly easy to recognize. What is more difficult is the relationship with someone who claims to love you but there are "red flags" that indicate that this is not a safe or healthy place to be. Some of the red flags include:

- *Physical assault* – even when it's "minor" (pushing, pinching, being restrained) and even when the person is extremely apologetic afterwards.

- *Physical abuse* – any kind of personal touching after you have made clear that it is unwanted by you. If you feel at all uncomfortable being physically close with someone, you have the right to say no and it should be respected – you don't need to have any other reason.

- *Verbal abuse* – being called names, belittling or humiliating comments, threats, yelling, a lack of respect for your decisions with regard to your own behavior (including your sexual choices).

- *Emotional abuse* – moodiness, one minute friendly, the next minute cold or angry, you are to blame for any problems, talking about belonging to each other, possessive, excluding and separating from friends or family, controlling how you dress and where you go.

What to do: Make sure that there are other people in your life, that there are times when you are able to be on your own, with your own friends, pursuing your own interests. Love does not mean having to share everything.

A relationship does not have to be all bad for it to be unhealthy. As with many other aspects of ourselves and our lives, there is likely to be a mixture of feelings. But if you are not able to be yourself, if you are being controlled or hurt by someone else, talk to someone you trust and ask their opinion. Don't isolate yourself.

Make sure there is a safe place you can get to easily if you need to talk, are frightened, or don't feel safe. Always have access to some money for yourself.

# CHAPTER 8

# Nuts and bolts of art techniques

Expressive art relates to paint, collage, any type of media which allows direct and spontaneous self-expression. In my experience, many very capable mental health professionals don't know where to start buying materials for art activities. While I am a strong believer in inventiveness in creative activities, I do believe good quality materials and the right tools make life easier and more enjoyable. The objective of this section of the book is to make the processing of buying and setting up materials for different crafts as simple as possible.

For specific and complex projects, there are better books available in craft shops – detailed, accompanied with pictures, and good value for money. Step-by-step instructions are attractive but can put a dent in imagination, inventiveness, spontaneity, and genuine expression, a central goal to these activities. After discussion of a theme and possible techniques, try to keep instructions to a minimum. Two rules should be to look after tools and clean up afterward.

It is always nice to produce pieces pleasing to the eye but the objective is not to be sophisticated or clever. It is really very easy to demystify art-related techniques so that they don't crush spontaneity and creativity, dominate a session, or turn the event into a new set of rules. Here are some basics.

## Wrapping technique

Paint on paper can sometimes look unfinished, even messy. This simple process finishes each piece and allows it to be used in different ways.

1.  Use an empty "frame" to roam over the finished piece of artwork and see it in frame. Sometimes a very attractive corner can be found, or an area which most effectively depicts the "message" or something to be kept.

2.  Cut the piece out, allowing for extra width and length of about 1 cm or half an inch.

3.  Place the finished artwork face down on a clean surface (ensuring the paint is thoroughly dry first).

4.  On top of the back of the artwork, center a piece of cardstock, cardboard, balsa wood, or sturdy surface, the size and shape of the desired finished work. This is the central, stablizing form for the artwork and will not be seen later.

5.  Fold and bend the sides around the stabilizing form. Fold corners diagonally, trimming if there is excess bulk – adhere on the back with glue stick (fast drying). Wrap each side to the back of the card and attach with a glue stick. The finished piece should have the desired artwork wrapped around the cardstock, leaving an unfinished back.

Pieces of wrapped cardstock can be finished by:

- covering the back with another piece of same-size paper or cloth.

- attaching and gluing the wrapped piece to another structure such as a box, effectively covering the unfinished back and neatly finishing the box with the artwork.

- gluing two unfinished backs together, perhaps securing ribbons or "hinges" that connect a series of wrapped doubles, effectively making a "screen" or accordion-type booklet.


## Books, journals, and cards

Constructing simple books or journals is helpful to collect and present different perspectives of the same theme in a cohesive manner, reinforcing principles and giving an importance that may be lost if they are not "brought together."

- A collection of "leaves" of the same size can be fastened together in one corner in a way that allows them to pivot like a fan.

- A book may remain a collection of looseleafs, contained in a box or tin which, itself, is part of the design process.

- Accordion books may or not be closed with a fastener. They may be folded or attached with a kind of hinge, as described in the "wrapping technique" above (Figure 8.1).

- A book might be folded up, like a compressed box.

- More conventional "books" can be made up of folded paper or single sheets, hole punched, and bound in different ways (Figure 8.2).

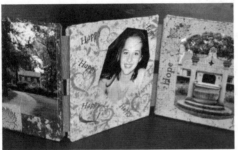

*Figure 8.1 Completed accordion book*

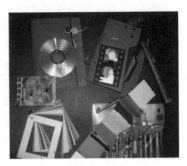

*Figure 8.2 Card making*

## Expressing self

Self-awareness is the most important theme to address and provides the basic foundation from which changes can be made. Self-awareness is not just about self-concept and image but also relevant to issues that arise during a week (awareness of feelings and role in argument with mother), which may potentially arise in the future (awareness of fear in reluctance to go to college), and feelings that are motivating behavior (awareness of what feelings occur around losing control). Self-awareness is about past, present, and future, about feelings.

Over a period of time most people find themes that they repeat and develop in one way or another. However, the most basic and spontaneous way to explore self is by painting feelings, from the heart. Paper and paint can be used again and again, each time producing different results and subsequent discussion, depending on "happy accidents," mood of the day, interaction with others in the group, and so on. Many activities in this book are to maintain interest and motivation through variety, but do not underestimate the following exercise which can be used again and again with minor variations. Dating work that is kept is very helpful in identifying progress and patterns.

Use a surface which is clear, with convenient access to paint, water, and a variety of brushes; a comfortable seat and appropriate space; sink, good lighting, temperature, and conducive background noise.

Relax, either through a guided meditation or a few minutes to inhale deeply and consciously release physical tension. Make this time a punctuation point, a time to detach from outside conditions, to focus inwardly, perhaps with eyes closed, paying attention to feelings, "pictures," colors, forms that present themselves to the mind's eye.

With eyes open again, look at the colors and brushes available. Choose a color or brush that is pleasing, without too much thought. Use the brushes and paints to make marks, shapes, lines, textures, one color, or a combination. Work out from a center or let each line take on a direction and life of its own. There may need to be some encouragement to be spontaneous and take risks – to paint with heart, not mind.

The focus throughout should be on what is felt rather than thoughts about the finished product. Play with instinct. Respond to what grows on the paper as a conversation would unfold. Respond with shapes and lines and colors. There are no rules and the piece is finished only when the person feels it is so.

Don't think or worry about the emerging image. There is always another piece of paper and more paint. Sometimes a sense of completion or resolution isn't experienced until a series of works have been completed, each piece developing the theme further. Sometimes the theme is developed only when the individual looks at it afterward, or is discussing what they were feeling rather than what was produced. Very often a theme does not even become conscious until it has been expressed a number of times, in different ways.

## Collage

Collages are recommended a great deal in this book. That's because they have the most potential to use a variety of materials, can be highly personalized with no more technical ability than being able to apply glue to paper. They can be simple, sophisticated, masculine, feminine, decorative pictures or applied to something practical (a useful three-dimensional collage). Many people prefer to take readymade templates, punches, die cuts, photographs, and pictures and rearrange them. This is fine – the projection and interpretation will say more than the finished project.

If there is a desire to be more definitive in a theme but uncertainty about how to proceed, read again the section on associative thinking. This gives a good foundation for any personalized exploration and is ideal for collage. Begin with a theme – "My family" or "Asperger's Syndrome" or "Happy memories." Let your mind flow, close your eyes, and take note of images that present themselves. Go through photographs, remember the smells and tastes and touches and colors. Look through magazines – do some pictures "jump out" and remind you of things you'd forgotten? Given the opportunity, the mind has a way of directing attention to that which is important to you.

When you've made many associations of thoughts, memories, and sensory experiences, consider how you might suggest some of them and "cross-reference." For example, could a sharp pain be suggested by sharp edges; happiness by a flower; sadness by a color? Symbols are personal and don't have to be understood by others or explained. Your thoughts and feelings might suggest materials to use (reflective thoughts – mirror) or materials that you consider or touch or come across might bring to mind one of your associations (the stamp of a frame can be used to frame a picture of the "happy me").

If "growth" is one of the ideas that emerge from your associations, explore all the things that you associate with growth: the color green, leaves, trees, yardstick. Any of these can be introduced through stamps, cut outs, stencils, paint, collaged shapes. Let's look just at the opportunities that arise with paper right now.

Imagine the variety of leaves you could make with paper – shredded, painted, printed, clipped, layered, turned, sewn, cut carefully, handmade paper, soft and crushed, hard and folded, corrugated, photographs of leaves, envelopes containing leaves – and that's just the paper. Now there are the colors. An envelope may suggest communication to some (was writing a part of your growth), secrets to another (secrets associated with growth). Creativity is interpretation – combining familiar elements in novel ways.

Papers for painting are briefly covered below. Having a "bank" of different papers is invaluable. They should come in a range of thicknesses and colors. The heaviest card can be bent with scoring tools if necessary, and can be used as a background. The lightest can be tissue or handmade paper and may even be transparent. Collage pieces can be cut with scissors or torn – pictures and print from magazines or made with paint, stamps, natural materials.

Collage doesn't have to be the haphazard shapes traditionally thought of. It can also be symmetrical in squares or rectangles (imagine a Persian carpet effect) or a circle (mandala). A mosaic or tile effect can be used. Collage can also be three-dimensional, using papers that easily flex such as the handmade papers, and can be glued down to another object such as a ball or lamp. White glue is reasonably priced, easily manipulated and cleaned up, and dries clear.

Collage can incorporate found objects, all of the media described below, and things you pick up in the park. Three dimensions can be introduced with pieces of metal, slices of sponge or wood, fabrics, corrugated paper, beads, wheels, wire – the list is endless. A box in the middle of the table of an assortment of odds and ends will broaden possibilities for creativity. Lay the materials/objects/ elements out on a board and rearrange them. If desired, the finished image can be given unity with a border, or repeated color, texture, or theme. (See Figure 8.3.)

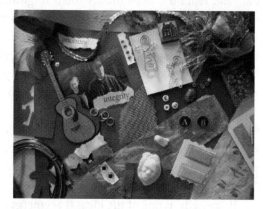

*Figure 8.3 Collage*

## Paint

The most economic and practical paints to use are one of the brands of folk art or acrylic paint. These come in a wide variety of colors (so color mixing doesn't waste a lot of time and paint), the bottles are small so spills are minimal, and they can be bought very cheaply at craft shops. Folk paint is also opaque (not transparent) which covers well, at a nice consistency, and dries quickly which is important if art work is to be carried home.

Watercolor paints are transparent and can be used for more translucent effects. They require a better quality, more expensive paper and will not be absorbed by the photocopy paper or seen on colored paper. There are a lot of cheap watercolor paints available but I would suggest a better grade for a more pleasant sensory experience for older group members. Interesting brushes and a quality watercolor paint will improve performance and enjoyment to the point that it is well worth the extra expense.

Oil paints are wonderful to use but have a strong smell and take too long to dry to be practical. There are additives, however, that can be added to waterbased paints for an oil consistency, texture, and effect. Keep an eye on new products in your craft shop or be on the mailing list for art supply catalogues. New innovations are constantly introduced to the market. Having a variety of materials available will make the art process a great more interesting and engaging for group members, especially those who wouldn't normally have access to them.

"Important" paintings can be finished through framing or laminating. They can be elaborated upon by making them into mosaics, transferring them onto mouse pads (computer transfer paper from office supply stores), and so on.

## Textured painting

Textured painting can be introduced with dyed sawdust, coffee grounds, or sand. The textured materials can have glue added to them and then be painted directly onto paper. Alternatively, glue can be applied first and the textured material shaken onto it afterward. Stamps can be used to apply glue in desired shapes – it is advisable to wash the stamps immediately afterward.

## Altered art

Altered art is very versatile for individualized craft. Books, cigar boxes, any three-dimensional shapes are interesting because of the opportunity to express layers, inside and outside, exposed and hidden, etc. The basic "bones" for these projects can be picked up at a reasonable cost at craft and dollar stores, or second-hand shops. Look for interesting shapes, the basis for a three-dimensional collage. They can be cut, glued together, added to and taken away, embellished and painted – endless possibilities.

For example, for altered books, take discarded, thick, hardcovered books and treat them like a solid box. Cut or tear a hole or various spaces out of the middle of the pages, leaving the edges intact. Glue what remains of the pages together, leaving spaces (an empty box, the front cover acting as a lid) for further development of a theme. Add paint, paper, collage, photographs, personal items, and embellishments.

Use finished pieces of art projects (paint, stamping, collage) to cover the box or book. The three dimensions give opportunities to express self in different ways to two dimensions (layers, hidden parts, etc.). The space within also allows incorporation of three-dimensional objects.

Still on the potential of three dimensions, simplify the art-making process by providing a container that can be covered, allowing the focus to be on the cover rather than the construction. Possibilities include an assortment of boxes and containers, tins, tubes. Allowing group members to choose from a variety of objects offers an opportunity to express a size, shape, or material that is preferred or inspiring, a design that is simplistic, eclectic, or sophisticated.

Useful names can be given to covered containers such as a desk hold-all, purse, tote or basket, cake box, or flower pot. More ideas are below. The finished product is not as important as the opportunity it gives to express a theme such as:

- Myself as a container
- Myself as an imaginary animal
- My friendships
- My sister/brother/teacher
- Having Asperger's Syndrome.

## Clay

Traditional clay products were not easily accessed or used because of the need for a kiln and the water content and messiness made cleaning up a nightmare. New products easily available through general craft suppliers allow clay to be used and oven baked with minimal effort, expense, or time-consuming fussiness. It is a colorful, tactile, versatile, and popular medium and useful for stamping, shaping, painting, sculpting.

## Sculpture

Three-dimensional shapes can be carved or constructed (Figure 8.4). An economical approach to construction is forming a basic shape with a cheap flexible material such as foam, wire, or cooking foil and then wrapping with fabric or paper strips and pieces. Basic shapes bought from craft shops (wooden/plastic boxes, clay pots, tin items) can also be modified or embellished. A company called Dazian (http://www.dazian.com)

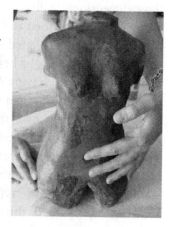

*Figure 8.4 Sculpture*

supplies theater and opera companies with costume materials and produces a thick fabric which can be draped and shaped, set with a heat gun and then painted. It can be used for large-scale works (life-size puppets, costumes, sculpture).

## Stamping

Lino cuts, stencils, potatoes, ready-made rubber stamps, and soap can be used to make impressions. The difficulty level varies slightly but they all operate on the principle of applying paint to paper (or fabric, wood, surfaces) with an individualized utensil. Some require sharp instruments (lino cuts, soap) and should be used appropriate to maturity level. Ready-made stamps are convenient but there is a danger of the individual using ready-made designs instead of their own creativity.

## Oil and chalk pastels

Pastels come in sticks and are very effective on black or colored paper and card. The chalk may smudge but can be fixed (between layers and when finished) with a fixative or hairspray. Take sprays outside if possible, or well away from the main working area. Their fumes fill a room quickly and can be dangerous. Chalk pastels are more expensive than oils but last for a long time. They can also be used on mixed media such as clay.

## Fabric

After paper, fabric is one of the cheapest and most versatile of craft materials. It doesn't have to be a "feminine" craft, especially if the print has a masculine theme, or it is used as a construction material (stretch, staple, glue onto other objects, use as a covering for a lamp, box, book cover, mix with a stiffener to use as a sculptural material). Fabric comes with wonderful colors so it is ideal as a collage material. Instead of using glue, use iron-on, double-sided fusing tape or fusible web. Ask at a fabric supply shop what they recommend for adhering two pieces of fabric together with no sewing.

Fabric collages are an alternative to paper collages and are no more difficult – as long as they won't be thrown in a washing machine. Fabric collages can be made into simple quilts, hangings, bags, personalized t-shirts. Small fabric pockets or bags can be used to carry mobile telephones. Personalize through paint, fused fabric, pens, etc., add drawstrings to be carried around the neck (Figure 8.5).

Fabric paints, dyes, crayons, and pens are invaluable because of their easiness to use and ability to be washed. A company called Dharma Trading Co. can be recommended for their products and have a comprehensive catalogue (http://www.dharma trading.com). Their products include a variety of fabrics and clothing ready to be painted or dyed, dye sticks, fabric paints, pens and crayons, books, markers, kits, tools, and inkjet transfer products.

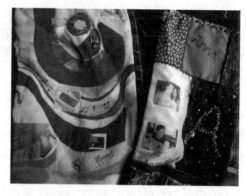

*Figure 8.5 Fabric collage*

## Inkjet transfer products

Technology and computers have opened up new worlds for the amateur artist. This is an ideal craft to explore for the Asperger artist. Graphic computer programs have endless possibilities for image manipulation, which can then be transferred to all manner of materials – from computer transfer sheets to fabric, clay, metal, wood. It is one of the most effective ways of individualizing art – apply personal photographs to multidimensional and functional objects. Some excellent books are available to develop this craft further and office and craft supply stores carry a variety of suitable inkjet transfer sheets.

## Metal

Craft stores supply a range of metals – mesh, strips with adhesive, sheets to be embossed. Hardware stores are treasure chests for metal in different shapes (bolts, discs, springs, cups, sheets) for three-dimensional collages. Plain can be transformed to colorful with a coat of metal spray paint. Embossing metals lend themselves to a variety of projects, in different metallic colors and weights. Wire is also available on spools for tying and constructing three-dimensional shapes and springs.

## Combination exercises – theme in the product

The effectiveness of expressive therapy is usually found in the process – the use of art as a tool to realize and express emotional issues and experiences. The expressive process can also offer catharsis value. Sometimes, however, the product itself can be a tool to explore and develop issues and themes. A box might be symbolic of self, a quilt might offer a structure for a story. An advantage to combining medium or constructing something like a box or quilt is also that the complexity and continuity will bring results that one-session exercises may not. Problem solving also becomes a tool, drawing on creativity, insight, and subconscious resources to make links and connections.

Although the value of paint on paper or collage cannot be underestimated, it may not be inspiring week after week. In the interests of keeping thoughts fresh and participants engaged, it is useful to combine materials such as metal and clay, or fabric and wood, or paint and glass (Figure 8.6). It is useful to suggest that a painting or collage be used as decoupage or applied to a sturdier surface to construct a box or CD case. It also suits the pragmatic, practical nature of the Asperger individual to produce a finished item.

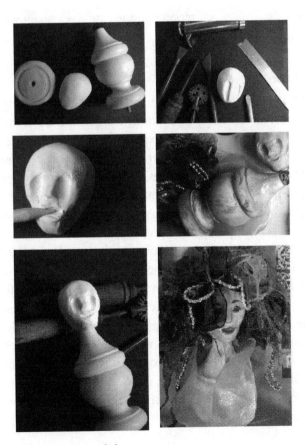

*Figure 8.6 Doorstop lady*

Ideas for simple items to build or buy and personalize with art include the following:

| | | |
|---|---|---|
| • beads | • desk organizers | • mouse pad |
| • biscuit tins | • door name plate | • old objects |
| • books | • frames | • pen covers |
| • bottles | • jewelry | • photo album cover |
| • "business" card | • journal | • pillow |
| • cards | • keyring | • plant container |
| • carry bag | • lantern | • puppets and dolls |
| • carved candle | • magnets | • quilt |
| • CD container | • mask | • scrapbook |
| • cigar box | • mobile phone case | • shadowbox picture |
| • craft wood | • mosaics | • tiles |

## Venue and tools

Environment is important. Adults who have participated in groups with me have often commented that the warmth and friendliness of the space contributed significantly to a positive experience. The environment was not anything out of the ordinary. However, there was a casual "homey" feeling, color on the walls, lots of space, cookies, and the coffee pot always hot. I have sometimes put posters and proverbs on walls to add to a sense of warmth, nothing is "precious," and corners are set up for people to work on the floor if they so desire. There may be a lot of preparation for art activities, but there is no fussing in the group itself over details, problems, spills. This is not a place to teach art. The focus is on the psychological comfort of the individual.

Ideal conditions include a room with at least enough space for a long or round table, chairs that allow for space between them (sometimes there is a need to stand up to work on something), and space to easily walk behind the chairs. A separate smaller table such as a card table can be used for heat guns, iron, or embossing tool if used (next to a wall with an outlet for electricity). The room will also need storage space, good ventilation, good lighting especially on dark and winter days, an easily accessed sink, a floor that doesn't need to be fussed over.

You will be surprised how many times water containers need to be refilled. Clean water is one of those small but important details that should not be forgotten. Heaviness of water containers is necessary to avoid spills. Paper – newsprint, butcher paper, photocopy paper, brown paper, card, colored pads of paper, wall paper, or the back of wrapping paper – should be readily available. Smaller pieces save waste and encourage use of different types.

In the middle of the table have at least two containers of assorted brushes. Don't be too cheap on brushes. The tactile pleasure that comes from the process of art is very much connected to the quality of the brushes. Have a variety of sizes and shapes available. Show group members different effects of different brushes and how to use them. For example, a scribbler can produce a very delicate "writing" stroke, an angle brush can have each end dipped in a different color to produce a shaded effect. Show group members how to keep brushes clean (provide a water container with serrated base) and expect them to clean them at the end of each session.

Some individuals will prefer some media over others. Some might not think of using something unless it is right in front of them and suggests itself. Encourage mixing up media – rules should be broken, alternative ways of making art encouraged. Encourage use of different materials for their tactile qualities.

Depending on the craft, other very helpful tools to have on hand include:

- scissors – include some with patterned blades (Fiskars); mark if for fabric or metal use only

- clear plastic boxes and bags so contents can be identified without being opened

- hole punches

- equipment for making words – alphabet punch, letters, label maker

- pencils, pens, markers, crayons – all colors, thicknesses, and textures

- glue sticks and white glue

- sewing kit, cottons, ribbons, all manner of things for threading

- rulers, set squares, shape templates

- small hammer and solid surface for pounding/punching/cutting

- die cut machine – although this is an initial expense it is extremely useful in saving preparation time and standardizing sizes (Figure 8.7)

- rubber stamps – can be used as themes in themselves or as texture, background, and borders

- ink pads in a variety of colors, and I have found a pad specifically for use with metal invaluable

- stencils, punches, embossing tools, tools to use specifically with metal or fabric

- heat gun for embossing

- newspapers (for supporting stamping, cutting, painting), rags (clean up), paper towels (wiping brushes), paper plates for throw away palettes, rubbish bags.

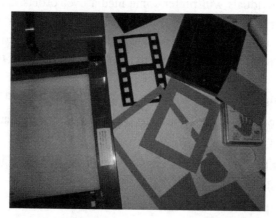

*Figure 8.7 Die cutting*

# VIA Classification of Character Strengths

These are the 24 strengths that are measured by the Values In Action Institute (VIA) Signature Strengths Survey. The names and descriptions of the strengths are taken from *Character Strengths and Virtues: A Handbook and Classification* (Peterson and Seligman 2004). The earlier versions used in *Authentic Happiness* (Seligman 2002) are in italics.

## Wisdom and knowledge
Cognitive strengths that entail the acquisition and use of knowledge.

1.  Creativity (originality, ingenuity). Thinking of novel and productive ways to do things; includes artistic achievement but is not limited to it.

    *Creativity, ingenuity, and originality – Thinking of new ways to do things is a crucial part of who you are. You are never content with doing something the conventional way if a better way is possible.*

2.  Curiosity (interest, novelty-seeking, openness to experience). Taking an interest in all of ongoing experience for its own sake; finding subjects and topics fascinating; exploring and discovering.

    *Curiosity and interest in the world – You are curious about everything. You are always asking questions, and you find all subjects and topics fascinating. You like exploration and discovery.*

3.  Open-mindedness (judgment, critical thinking). Thinking things through and examining them from all sides; not jumping to conclusions; being able to change one's mind in light of evidence; weighing all evidence fairly.

    *Judgment, critical thinking, and open-mindedness – Thinking things through and examining them from all sides are important aspects of who you are. You do not jump to conclusions, and you rely only on solid evidence to make your decisions. You are able to change your mind.*

4.  Love of learning. Mastering new skills, topics, and bodies of knowledge, whether on one's own or formally; obviously related to the

strength of curiosity but goes beyond it to describe the tendency to add systematically to what one knows.

*Love of learning – You love learning new things, whether in a class or on your own. You have always loved school, reading, and museums – anywhere and everywhere there is an opportunity to learn.*

5.    Perspective (wisdom). Being able to provide wise counsel to others; having ways of looking at the world that make sense to oneself and to other people.

     *Perspective (wisdom) – Although you may not think of yourself as wise, your friends hold this view of you. They value your perspective on matters and turn to you for advice. You have a way of looking at the world that makes sense to others and to yourself.*

## Courage

Emotional strengths that involve the exercise of will to accomplish goals in the face of opposition, external or internal.

6.    Bravery (valor). Not shrinking from threat, challenge, difficulty, or pain; speaking up for what is right even if there is opposition; acting on convictions even if unpopular; includes physical bravery but is not limited to it.

     *Bravery and valor – You are a courageous person who does not shrink from threat, challenge, difficulty, or pain. You speak up for what is right even if there is opposition. You act on your convictions.*

7.    Persistence (perseverance, industriousness). Finishing what one starts; persisting in a course of action in spite of obstacles; "getting it out the door"; taking pleasure in completing tasks.

     *Industry, diligence, and perseverance – You work hard to finish what you start. No matter the project, you "get it out the door" in timely fashion. You do not get distracted when you work, and you take satisfaction in completing tasks.*

8.    Integrity (authenticity, honesty). Speaking the truth but more broadly presenting oneself in a genuine way; being without pretense; taking responsibility for one's feelings and actions.

     *Honesty, authenticity, and genuineness – You are an honest person, not only by speaking the truth but by living your life in a genuine and authentic way. You are down to earth and without pretense; you are a "real" person.*

9.    Vitality (zest, enthusiasm, vigor, energy). Approaching life with excitement and energy; not doing things halfway or halfheartedly; living life as an adventure; feeling alive and activated.

*Zest, enthusiasm, and energy – Regardless of what you do, you approach it with excitement and energy. You never do anything halfway or halfheartedly. For you, life is an adventure.*

## Humanity

Interpersonal strengths that involve "tending" and "befriending" others.

10. Love. Valuing close relations with others, in particular those in which sharing and caring are reciprocated; being close to people.

    *Capacity to love and be loved – You value close relations with others, in particular those in which sharing and caring are reciprocated. The people to whom you feel most close are the same people who feel most close to you.*

11. Kindness (generosity, nurturance, care, compassion, altruistic love, "niceness"). Doing favors and good deeds for others; helping them; taking care of them.

    *Kindness and generosity – You are kind and generous to others, and you are never too busy to do a favor. You enjoy doing good deeds for others, even if you do not know them well.*

12. Social intelligence (emotional intelligence, personal intelligence). Being aware of the motives and feelings of other people and oneself; knowing what to do to fit in to different social situations; knowing what makes other people tick.

    *Social intelligence – You are aware of the motives and feelings of other people. You know what to do to fit in to different social situations, and you know what to do to put others at ease.*

## Justice

Civic strengths that underlie healthy community life.

13. Citizenship (social responsibility, loyalty, teamwork). Working well as a member of a group or team; being loyal to the group; doing one's share.

    *Citizenship, teamwork, and loyalty – You excel as a member of a group. You are a loyal and dedicated teammate, you always do your share, and you work hard for the success of your group.*

14. Fairness. Treating all people the same according to notions of fairness and justice; not letting personal feelings bias decisions about others; giving everyone a fair chance.

*Fairness, equity, and justice – Treating all people fairly is one of your abiding principles. You do not let your personal feelings bias your decisions about other people. You give everyone a chance.*

15.  Leadership. Encouraging a group of which one is a member to get things done and at the same time maintain good relations within the group; organizing group activities and seeing that they happen.

*Leadership – You excel at the tasks of leadership: encouraging a group to get things done and preserving harmony within the group by making everyone feel included. You do a good job organizing activities and seeing that they happen.*

## Temperance
Strengths that protect against excess.

16.  Forgiveness and mercy. Forgiving those who have done wrong; giving people a second chance; not being vengeful.

*Forgiveness and mercy – You forgive those who have done you wrong. You always give people a second chance. Your guiding principle is mercy and not revenge.*

17.  Humility/modesty. Letting one's accomplishments speak for themselves; not seeking the spotlight; not regarding one's self as more special than one is.

*Modesty and humility – You do not seek the spotlight, preferring to let your accomplishments speak for themselves. You do not regard yourself as special, and others recognize and value your modesty.*

18.  Prudence. Being careful about one's choices; not taking undue risks; not saying or doing things that might later be regretted.

*Caution, prudence, and discretion – You are a careful person, and your choices are consistently prudent ones. You do not say or do things that you might later regret.*

19.  Self-regulation (self-control). Regulating what one feels and does; being disciplined; controlling one's appetites and emotions.

*Self-control and self-regulation – You self-consciously regulate what you feel and what you do. You are a disciplined person. You are in control of your appetites and your emotions, not vice versa.*

## Transcendence
Strengths that forge connections to the larger universe and provide meaning.

20.  Appreciation of beauty and excellence (awe, wonder, elevation). Noticing and appreciating beauty, excellence, and/or skilled

performance in all domains of life, from nature to art to mathematics to science to everyday experience.

*Appreciation of beauty and excellence – You notice and appreciate beauty, excellence, and/or skilled performance in all domains of life, from nature to art to mathematics to science to everyday experience.*

21.  Gratitude. Being aware of and thankful for the good things that happen; taking time to express thanks.

*Gratitude – You are aware of the good things that happen to you, and you never take them for granted. Your friends and family members know that you are a grateful person because you always take the time to express your thanks.*

22.  Hope (optimism, future-mindedness, future orientation). Expecting the best in the future and working to achieve it; believing that a good future is something that can be brought about.

*Hope, optimism, and future-mindedness – You expect the best in the future, and you work to achieve it. You believe that the future is something that you can control.*

23.  Humor (playfulness). Liking to laugh and tease; bringing smiles to other people; seeing the light side; making (not necessarily telling) jokes.

*Humor and playfulness – You like to laugh and tease. Bringing smiles to other people is important to you. You try to see the light side of all situations.*

24.  Spirituality (religiousness, faith, purpose). Having coherent beliefs about the higher purpose and meaning of the universe; knowing where one fits within the larger scheme; having beliefs about the meaning of life that shape conduct and provide comfort.

*Spirituality, sense of purpose, and faith – You have strong and coherent beliefs about the higher purpose and meaning of the universe. You know where you fit in the larger scheme. Your beliefs shape your actions and are a source of comfort to you.*

# Music List

Thank you to Jenny Scott and Kim Dunphy for this extract from their book *Freedom to Move* (2003).

## World music
Saltwater Band, *Gapu Damurrun*, Skinnyfish Music, www.skinnyfishmusic.com.au (1998).
Lively rhythmic tracks by Australian aboriginal band.

Minjarah, *Tribal Trance*, Tribal World Music Distribution (1999).
Excellent selection from flowing to strong rhythms.

Various artists, *Afro Latino*, Putumayo World Music (1998).
Rhythmic and joyful African and Latin music.

Mickey Hart, *Planet Drum*, Rykodisc (1991).
Great drumming music and vocals.

Café del Mar, *Arias 2: New Horizon*, Café del Mar Music, Ibiza (1999).
Mellow and subdued, gentle and haunting.

Gypsy Soul, *New Flamenco*, Narada Productions (1999).
Flowing rhythms: great to get the arms and legs moving.

Mikis Theodorakis, *Zorba* (soundtrack), EMI (2000).
Modern disco-style Greek music for circle and traveling dances.

Various artists, *A Jewish Odyssey*, Putumayo World Music (1998).
"Dancing on Water: Meron Nigun," *Klezmania*, Oystralia, www.klezmania.com.au, Shanachie (1997).
Lively Israeli and Klezmer-style music.

## Classical/mellow
*For stretches/quieter warm-up activities*
Alice Gomez, *Flute Dreams*, TalkingTaco Music (1994).
Compositions that reflect the cultural heritage of the native peoples of the Americas.

Track 5, Marisa Robles, *The World of the Harp*, Universal/Decca (1992).
Ambient harp music, ideal for a slowing down activity.

*Improvisation*

Steve Falk, *The Marimba Project*, sfalk@iprimus.com.au (2000).
Interesting free-form marimba music, great for nature/environment/sea themes.

Jean-Michel Jarr, *Oxygene*, Jarr Records (1993).

David Bowie, *A Space Odyssey*, Rhino/Wea (2001).
Ambient, otherworldly.

Cirque du Soleil, *Collections*, RCA Victor (1998).
Magical.

Carl Orff, *Carmina Burana*.
Good for eliciting strong movement.

Mozart, Clarinet Concerto in A Major, *The Great Dream Classics*, Delta (1998).
Good for eliciting light movements.

Balanesque Quartet, *Possessed*, Mute Records (1992).
Sharp, definite, industrial.

Bert Kempfert, *Roses*, tracks 10–14, Taragon (2001).
Playful.

Sidney Berlin Ragtime Band, *Doop Doop*, Liberation Records (1994).
Energetic, fun, and wacky music good for traveling and spontaneity.

*Relaxation/resting*

Handel, Water Music, *Great Classics Series*, Delta Music (1994).
Flowing, watery.

Daniel Scott, *The Celtic Spirit*, Classic Fox Records (2000).
Also available with accompanying book of poems.

K.C. Wang, *Chinese Bamboo Flute Songs*, Dex Audio (1996).
Lyrical Chinese-style flute music.

Enya, *Paint the Sky With Stars*, Warner Music (1997).
Hauntingly beautiful melodies, Irish-Gaelic singer.

Nomade, *Hussein El Masry*, Iris Musique Productions France (1997).
Evocative Middle Eastern music.

# References

American Psychiatric Association (2000) *Diagnostic and Statistical Manual of Mental Disorders, Fourth Edition, Text Revision*. Washington, DC: APA.

Attwood, T. (1998) *Asperger's Syndrome: A Guide for Parents and Professionals*. London: Jessica Kingsley Publishers.

Beutler, L.E., Clarkin, J.F. and Bongar, B. (2000) *Guidelines for the Systematic Treatment of the Depressed Patient*. New York: Oxford University Press.

Boone, B. (1989) "Pitch synchrony in *Live with Regis and Kathie Lee* dialogue." California State University, Fresno Department of Music (unpublished paper).

Buzan, T. and Buzan, B. (1993) *The Mind Map Book*. New York: Plume.

Cohen, J.J. (1999) "Social and emotional learning past and present: A psychoeducational dialogue." In J. Cohen (ed) *Educating Minds and Hearts*. New York: Teachers College Press.

Cohen, J.J. (ed) (2001) *Caring Classrooms/Intelligent Schools*. New York: Teachers College Press.

Csikszentmihalyi, M. (1990) *Flow: The Psychology of Optimal Experience*. New York: Harper & Row.

Csikszentmihalyi, M. (1996) *Creativity: Flow and the Psychology of Discovery and Invention*. New York: HarperCollins.

Csikszentmihalyi, M. (1997) *Finding Flow in Everyday Life*. New York: Basic Books.

Csikszentmihalyi, M. and Csikszentmihalyi, I.S. (1988) *Optimal Experience: Psychological Studies of Flow in Consciousness*. Cambridge: Cambridge University Press.

Csikszentmihalyi, M., Rathunde, K. and Whalen, S. (1997) *Talented Teenagers: The Roots of Success and Failure*. Cambridge: Cambridge University Press.

de Bono, E. (1990) *I am Right: You are Wrong*. New York: Viking.

de Bono, E. (1993) *Teach Your Child How to Think*. London: Penguin.

Douglis, C. (1987) "The beat goes on: Social rhythms underlie all our speech and actions." *Psychology Today*, November, 40.

Dunphy, K. and Scott, J. (2003) *Freedom to Move*. Sydney: MacLennan and Petty.

Fling, H. (1973) *Marionettes: How to Make Them and Work Them*. New York: Dover.

Frankl, V.E. (1997) *Man's Search for Meaning*. New York: Washington Square Press.

Fredrickson, B. (1998) "What good are positive emotions?" *Review of General Psychology 2*, 300–319.

Fredrickson, B. (2001) "The role of positive emotions in Positive Psychology: The broaden-and-build theory of positive emotion." *American Psychologist 56*, 218–226.

Fullerton, A., Stratton, J., Coyne, P. and Gray, C. (1996) *Higher Functioning Adolescents and Young Adults with Autism: A Teacher's Guide*. Austin, TX: Pro-ed.

Grandin, T. (1995) *Thinking in Pictures*. New York: Doubleday.

Grandin, T. (1999) *Visual Thinking of a Person with Autism*. Arlington, TX: Future Horizons.

Gray, C. (1994) *Comic Strip Conversations*. Jenison: Jenison Public Schools.

Gray, C. (2000) *The New Social Story Book*. Arlington, TX: Future Horizons.

Jackson, L. (2002) *Freaks, Geeks and Asperger Syndrome: A User Guide to Adolescence.* London: Jessica Kingsley Publishers.

Koch, K. and Students of P.S.61 in New York City (1970) *Wishes, Lies, and Dreams: Teaching Children to Write Poetry.* New York: HarperCollins.

Ledgin, N.L.M. (2002) *Asperger's and Self Esteem: Insight and Hope through Famous Role Models.* Arlington, TX: Future Horizons.

MacGregor, S. (1994) *Students Step to Success.* Lindfield: CALM.

Mugno, D. and Rosenblitt, D. (2001) "Helping emotionally vulnerable children: Moving toward an empathic orientation in the classroom." In J.J. Cohen (ed) *Caring Classrooms/ Intelligent Schools.* New York: Teachers College Press.

Murray, J. (2000) *Religious Belief and Behavior for African Americans: Relationship to Health?* Paper presented at the American Psychological Association Annual Conference, San Francisco.

Ortiz, J.M. (1997) *The Tao of Music: Sound Psychology.* Maine: Weiser Books.

Peterson, C. and Seligman, M.E.P. (2004) *Character Strengths and Virtues: A Handbook and Classification.* Oxford: Oxford University Press.

Rathunde, K. (2001) "Family context and the development of undivided interest: A longitudinal study of family support and challenge and adolescents' quality of experience." *Applied Developmental Science 5,* 3, 158–171.

Reivich, K. and Shatte, A. (2002) *The Resilience Factor.* New York: Random House.

Roberts, J. (1999) "Beyond words: The power of rituals." In D.J. Wiener (ed) *Beyond Talk Therapy.* Washington, DC: American Psychological Association.

Rowitz, L. and Jurkowski, E. (1995) "The myths and realities of depression and Down Syndrome." In L. Nadel and D. Rosenthal (eds) *Down Syndrome: Living and Learning in the Community.* Proceedings of the Fifth International Down Syndrome Conference. New York: Wiley-Liss.

Schaffer, R.J., Jacokes, L.E., Cassily, J.F., Greenspan, S.I., Tuchman, R.F., and Stemmer, P.J. (2001) "Effect of interactive metronome training on children with ADHD." *American Journal of Occupational Therapy 55,* 2, 155–162.

Seligman, M.E.P. (2002) *Authentic Happiness.* New York: Free Press.

Standley, J. (1991) *Music Techniques in Therapy, Counseling, and Special Education.* Saint Louis: MMB Music.

Walsh-Stewart, R. (2002) "Combined efforts: Increasing social-emotional communication with children with autistic spectrum disorder using psychodynamic music therapy and division TEACCH communication programme." In A. Davies and E. Richards (eds) *Music Therapy and Group Work: Sound Company.* London: Jessica Kingsley Publishers.

Willey, L.H. (1999) *Pretending to be Normal: Living with Asperger's Syndrome.* London: Jessica Kingsley Publishers.

# Subject index

# Author index